Finding the JOY in Alzheimer's is a breath of fresh air in the heavy atmosphere of Alzheimer's disease. The lovingly told humorous stories and anecdotes prove once again that laughter is good medicine, a welcome tonic to weary AD caregivers.

B.J. FitzRay, Author
Alzheimer's Activities: Hundreds of Activites for Men and Women with Alzheimer's Disease

Avadian has selected stories that fill the heart with joy, laughter, hope, and understanding of the essence of living with Alzheimer's.

Patricia Weber
ForeWord Magazine

... a comforting, spiritually healing book filled with touches of wry humor and a serious understanding of the difficulties of Alzheimer's, and how important it is to find and treasure wondrous moments when caring for someone afflicted with this debilitating neurological disease. *Finding The Joy In Alzheimer's* ... was written to bolster the souls and spirits of those charged with caregiving responsibilities for loved ones suffering from the ravages of Alzheimer's. As such, it emphatically succeeds in its mission and intention.

Midwest Book Review

I read "Joy" and found it wonderful! I laughed and I cried. It's a book to help people see the big picture within the smaller episodes or vignettes.

Sara E. Parrish, Author
How to Be a Parent FOR Your Parent

Finding the JOY in Alzheimer's captured the thoughts and memories I have of my twin sister, Janette Shulman. I was especially touched by the poem "A Hug, a Tender Touch," by Marian Summers. After years of joy and laughter, it is heartbreaking to see her in the throws of Alzheimer's disease. But my thoughts are of gratitude for the many happy years that we have had, and now we take it one day at a time, never knowing what tomorrow may bring.

Janice Greenhouse

Finding the JOY in Alzheimer's might be a difficult task, but Brenda Avadian brings joy and humor to everything in life, as she's done with this joyful, heartwarming book.

Jim Barnes, Managing Editor
Independent Publisher Online
www.independentpublisher.com

Witnessing my mother's abilities and personality wither away from Alzheimer's has been difficult. Comfort and advice from friends, family, and the medical community has helped, and so has reading Brenda Avadian's brilliantly conceived and constructed book, *Finding the Joy in Alzheimer's*. Discovering what others have experienced and learned in similar circumstances—particularly, the heartfelt reflections of joy—has enabled me to see my mother and her disease in a new, brighter light. Highly recommended.

Lee Godden, Author
Zen Wise Selling

Finding the JOY in Alzheimer's made me realize that people can be funny without even noticing it. My grandmother didn't come up with as many funny things, but now I realize that other Alzheimer's victims do. I liked the story where the woman kept saying the same things over and over, like my grandma does.

Joel Center, Age 8

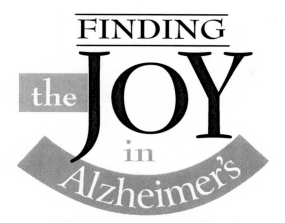

FINDING the JOY in Alzheimer's

CAREGIVERS SHARE
THE JOYFUL TIMES

BRENDA AVADIAN, MA
Author of *"Where's my shoes?"*
My Father's Walk Through Alzheimer's

NORTH STAR BOOKS
Pearblossom, California

We acknowledge the following individuals for permission to include their material. (Note: stories and photos by Brenda Avadian, MA are not included in this listing.)

Amazing Vision. Printed with permission from Debbie Center. ©1999 Debbie Center

Bad Hair Day. Printed with permission from Joan Fry. ©2001 Joan Fry

A Bedtime Story. Printed with permission from Marion Riley. ©2001 Marion Riley

Credits continued on p. 155

Library of Congress Publisher's Cataloging-in-Publication Data
Avadian, Brenda, MA
    Finding the joy in Alzheimer's: caregivers share the joyful times /
    Brenda Avadian, MA — Lancaster, CA: North Star Books, 2002.
       p.   ill.   cm.
    1. Health — Alzheimer's disease — Caregiving — Humor
    ISBN-13: 978-0-9632752-2-6
    ISBN-10: 0-9632752-2-4
    Library of Congress Control Number 2001117532

Third Printing 2010 (updated 2006)

Printed in the United States of America

NORTH STAR BOOKS
P. O. Box 589
Pearblossom, California 93553 U.S.A.
Telephone: 661.944.1130
E-mail: NSB@NorthStarBooks.com

*Dedicated to
the quiet majority of caregivers
who endure unimaginable sacrifices
to provide quality care
for their loved ones.*

Warning - Disclaimer

Contents

SECTION I
Who? What? Where?

SECTION II
Children Show the Way

SECTION III
Loving Couples

SECTION IV
Friends are Like Family

SECTION V
Celebrations

SECTION VI
The Birds and the Bees

SECTION VII
Discoveries in Nursing Homes

CONTENTS

Acknowledgments

As with any undertaking, real success rests not with the name on the cover but with everyone who selflessly shared their talents in order to complete this project. There are many who came forward to help. I thank each of them, because without them this book would not be in your hands right now.

First and most important are the contributors, who willingly told a part of their life story—the joy they found while enduring the challenge of caring for their loved ones.

Next are the caregivers, who share a unique understanding of the highs and lows of the caregiving journey and who can laugh heartily, despite the heartbreaks, knowing they have company. They say, "We laugh so we won't cry."

Then there are those who helped spread the word about our campaign to find the joy, including: adult day care centers; assisted living centers; *CareGiving Families;* the contributors themselves; geriatric assessment centers; nursing homes; *The Ribbon*; and the Alzheimer's Association—Greater Austin, Orange County, Riverside/San Bernardino Counties, Southern Nevada, and Ventura County.

Also, there are those who inspired this book's title, including the Ventura County office of the Alzheimer's Association, caregivers from the Lancaster Adult Day Health Care Support Group in Lancaster, California (formerly Visiting Nurse) and from the Antelope Valley Care Center's luncheon group including: Rosa Lee Boslar, Edith Pledger, Marion Riley, and Joe Shell.

And there is Carole Kelly, who arranges canine visits to the care center where my father lived, and other facilities, who said, "If they are polite, enjoy meeting and being touched by strangers, they may be potential therapy dogs." To learn more visit their website at www.therapydogs.com.

I am indebted to my editor and book designer, Mary Jo Zazueta of To the Point Solutions, whose eye for detail enables us to convey these JOYful stories clearly and attractively; and whose patience with me often goes beyond the call of duty.

I thank Julia Ryan of Design by Julia, who designed a fabulous cover, which is drawing rave reviews, and who, in a few short months, has grown to be my friend. In addition to sharing a passion for this project, Julia makes some of the BEST chocolate chip cookies I have eaten, rivaling those made by my husband, David. (Thank you, Mary Jo Jirik at Dunn+Associates for referring Julia.)

Also, two designers deserve mention. Although I did not have the opportunity to work with them, both did influence my ideas about this project: George Foster of Foster and Foster, Inc. and Pam Terry of Opus 1 Design.

Finally, trying to put together materials for a book with photos requires a degree of technical know-how (scanning, importing files, writing to CDs, etc.). David Borden, my husband, was quickly recruited as "Technical Support." This included many duties only a husband would lovingly perform for his wife. (I still smile thinking of this.)

CareGiver

Two words that come together
When you speak of someone
dear.
It is that special person
If you call, they're always near.

You'll see that in a "Care-
Giver"
Love comes from in their
Heart.
With loving hands and guid-
ance
They help each new day start.

Caring for the fragile soul,
Giving day to day.
They meet the needs of
loved ones
Spreading love along the way.

A gentle touch,
a helping hand,
A glow that makes you smile.
Always near to comfort
And go that extra mile.

They want no fame or glory,
And it puts their mind
at ease,
To know they've helped
a loved one
Deal with Alzheimer's disease.

So show a little kindness
To CareGivers across this
land.
You may be the one someday
Who needs a helping hand.

With Peace
and Understanding
Throughout the end of time.
There's someone who will
care for you
And make your spirit shine ...

The CareGiver ...

LORAINE YATES (WILLO)

13

Introduction

Is there JOY in Alzheimer's? During the three years I was developing my vision for this book I asked this question. People had varying reactions. Many stopped what they were doing, and seemed to really give the idea some thought. "Well, yeee-aaa-ah, I suppose there can be."

Actor David Hyde Pierce (Niles on *Frasier*) and activist for Alzheimer's causes, chuckled and admitted he could think of a number of JOYful experiences with his family (his father and grandfather had Alzheimer's). Then he added with a fiendish grin, "None that I could share!"

Others offered guidance when I volunteered what I was working on: "Don't do it because people may take it wrong. You might offend them." "How can there be joy in Alzheimer's?" several asked, including actress and Alzheimer's spokesperson Shelley Fabares.

Were they right?

My husband, David, and I had journeyed a bumpy and painful road with my father. Ironically, less of it had to do with caring for *him* than it did for his estate and dealing with family members. Despite the graveness of the disease, managing the details of a complicated estate, one accountant, six attorneys, and siblings with whom I am in contact only through attorneys—we managed to find the JOYs. Sometimes they were bittersweet, such as when my father expressed his wish to die and then changed his mind once breakfast was ready.

Other times, we smiled, chuckled, and even laughed during truly funny moments.

I planned to write about these JOYs because, despite the pain, we found reasons to laugh. Some of the JOYs were small and got smaller each day the disease took its toll. Still, they were JOYs and we grasped at them and treasured them as the disease took my father away piece by heartbreaking piece.

As I shared this project with other caregivers at support group meetings and during online chats, they enthusiastically embraced the idea. Some wanted to buy a copy of the book, while others offered their own stories. I encouraged them to put their stories in writing and to send them for possible inclusion in *Finding the JOY in Alzheimer's*.

I believe this project, which began as a solo journey, will touch many more lives, because the stories come from different perspectives—loving couples, children, grandchildren, siblings, and friends. The youngest contributor is ten years old and "the most life-experienced children" are in their eighties. Their JOYful stories span caregiving through the early stages to late stages of Alzheimer's disease.

An unexpected benefit caregivers received after writing their stories was a greater acceptance of the quality of care they gave to their loved ones. As they took the time to write and organize their thoughts, they wrote of the pleasant feelings they had in letting go of their intense feelings of guilt, sadness, and of being overwhelmed. They felt a newfound comfort in being able to write their heartfelt words on paper. Some, who initially wanted to be sure their stories would be included, echoed these sentiments in notes submitted with their stories. They didn't care if their stories weren't selected; they felt fortunate to reflect on the JOYful times with their loved ones.

Much to my surprise, most weren't even impressed that they could be a *published* author. I smile as I write this, because most of these contributors are not professional writers. They are caring for their loved ones day-to-day. They did not want to add writing to their already heavy burden of responsibilities. However, encouraged that their words may help others, they took time to write their stories. Many included their heartfelt struggles, pain, and the challenges of caring for a loved one. At the same time, they are learning to accept Alzheimer's for what it is; and they are *Finding the JOY* as they recount in the stories that follow.

This, in my opinion, is the greatest value. Although edited for publication, each story carries a message direct from the caregiver's heart.

It has been my pleasure to read their stories and the ones that continue to arrive for our next volume of *Finding the JOY in Alzheimer's*.

What follows is a prescription of JOY for you, the caregiver: When you feel overwhelmed, lost and alone, and the world rests its burden upon your shoulders, take *Finding the JOY in Alzheimer's*, open it, and read whatever story unfolds upon the pages before you, as that is the one you need. Read one a day and in a little over a month you should be well on your way to *Finding the JOY in Alzheimer's*.

SECTION I

Who? What? Where?

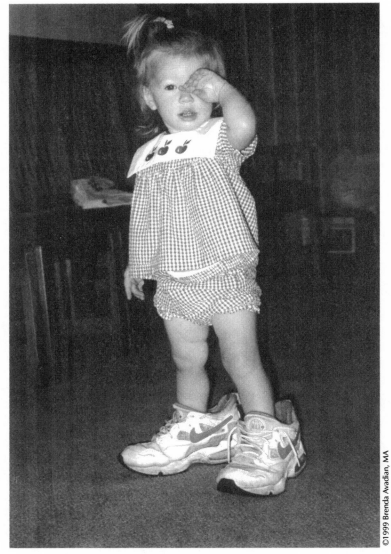

"Where's my shoes?"
Eleanor Borden, 18 months, wearing the author's shoes.

Alzheimer's disease is the most common cause of dementia (compared to other dementia-related diseases such as: Parkinson's, Lewy body, and vascular). Alzheimer's causes people to forget, to lose their sense of time and place. As the disease takes hold of nearly five million people in the U.S. alone, and an estimated twelve million worldwide, its victims become disoriented and unable to communicate or function physically. They can be vulnerable in a society that is still learning about this disease. Thanks to well-known celebrities—former President Ronald Reagan, David Hyde Pierce, Shelley Fabares, and others, the world is beginning to learn more about Alzheimer's.

Memory loss is commonly associated with Alzheimer's and with it comes the forgetting of friends and family members. Ironically, long-term memory stays in place longer than short-term memory. Many victims in their seventies and eighties recall things from forty years ago.

I often joked with other caregivers that my ninety-year-old father wanted to forget my siblings and me, when about three years ago his entire memory of our existence was wiped clean. He no longer remembered me, his "fellow Leo," who was born on his forty-ninth birthday.

"Who's the father?" depicts a victim's confusion about roles. Micah Leslie and Joan Fry write about similar experiences in " 'Damn, you're handsome!' " and "Bad Hair Day." And, sometimes they can't make sense of things we take for granted, like time, in "Making Sense of Time."

Yet there are lucid moments when they can perform normally. "Amazing Vision" is the story of Debbie Center's vision-impaired mother whose ability to read surprised her family. In "Whose Prosthesis is This Anyway?" Gil Lozano recounts a few fun and embarrassing adventures with his ninety-year old mother, who remembers that she has a prosthesis, and wants to use it, but claims it isn't hers.

As they forget and misplace things, people with Alzheimer's often think, "*They* are taking them." My father would go to great pains to hide his shaver, wallet, and other items of value, only to forget where he had hidden them. He'd then cry out, "*They* are taking my things!" Others misplace objects and think they are losing their minds, as is the case for Loraine Yates' mother in " 'I've got rocks in my head!' "

Most of all, people with Alzheimer's need a loving caregiver to protect them from harming themselves. Like children, they may unknowingly do things to hurt themselves. Loraine Yates shares an example in "Don't Eat the Yellow and Green Ones."

"What's the name of that disease where you forget ... ?"

In the years before my mother was diagnosed with Alzheimer's disease she asked me, "What's the name of that disease where you *forget* things? I can never *remember* what it's called."

DIANE BLAKE

"I've got rocks in my head!"

As caregivers of people with Alzheimer's, we hear things repeated over and over; sometimes it seems like a thousand times! The same questions asked and the same phrases spoken by our loved ones, who have no memory of saying them just two minutes ago! The one that will stick with me forever is: "I've got rocks in my head!"

My little mama was a collector. "Of what?" you ask. Rocks! For as long as I can remember, wherever we went as a family, Mama found a special rock that she would bring home. There were large rocks, tiny rocks, and rocks that sparkled and shined. You could find all the colors of the rainbow in her Rock Garden.

As the years passed and Mama moved from place to place, so did her rocks! When the time came that my little mama couldn't live on her own anymore, we moved her into our home—her and the rocks.

Mama sits for hours checking each groove, scratch, and shape in her rock collection. Since her memory is fading, we've labeled the rocks so that she can remember which part of the country they came from.

She often forgets to put them back on their special shelf, so we find "Palm Springs" in the bathroom, "Grand Canyon" on the kitchen counter, and "Colorado River" between the video tapes. But the night we found "Hawaii" in her bed was the night my little mama started saying, "Boy oh boy! I think I've got rocks in my head!"

LORAINE YATES (WILLO)

Amazing Vision

About a year ago I told Mom that part of the reason we were worried about her living alone was because her vision was so bad she might not be able to see what she was eating. For example, was it food or cleanser?

Of course, she thought I was nuts, so I proved it. I held up a liter of Pepsi® and asked her what it was.

She stared, and stared, and stared. Mom could not read the giant letters that spelled "Pepsi®." Then she turned the bottle around and said, "Oh yes, says here it has 100 calories and 0 grams of fat."

I about DIED.

She couldn't begin to read letters that were nearly one-and-a-half inches tall but she could make out the eighth-inch letters just fine! Then I handed her a Tombstone® pizza with two-inch letters and asked her what it was.

Again, she stared and stared. Nothing. Finally, she read the bottom. "Oh yes, it says 'KEEP FROZEN'."

Swell. Eighth-inch letters are okay, two-inch ones are not. Isn't that weird?

After the Pepsi® incident we both laughed as I said, "Good Mom, you have NO clue what you're pouring, but you know it has 100 calories and 0 grams of fat."

DEBBIE CENTER
Piano Teacher

"Damn, you're handsome!"

I was preparing for a speaking engagement and came downstairs in a shirt and tie, which is not my normal attire.

My mother looked at me strangely and inquired, "Are you my husband?"

"No," I replied.

"Are you my boyfriend?"

"No."

She remained still, and then said, "Damn, you're handsome!"

I awkwardly replied, "Well, thanks. I'll give you a hint. I get my good looks from my mom."

A big ol' grin spread across her face and she said, "I know now. You're my boy ... I love you."

MICAH J. LESLIE

Bad Hair Day

"Mom needs help," my sister-in-law announced the second I picked up the phone. "Dad's in bad shape."

"What kind of help does she need?" I asked, side-stepping the real question.

"Grocery shopping. Leaving him alone in the house while she gets her hair done."

"Can't she hire somebody to go grocery shopping?"

"How long has it been since you saw them?"

"John and I drove down a couple of months ago and took them to lunch."

"He's gotten worse. That's what Mom really needs—help with Dad."

I told her I'd talk to John.

The real question was one we had all tiptoed around for the past eighteen months: Did John's father have Alzheimer's?

Nelson was a big man with a salesman's outgoing manner. He was quick to offer help whenever he thought somebody needed it—waitresses, the mail carrier, someone standing in line at the bank. He adored children in particular, probably because he saw them as small, inarticulate people who could always use help.

The four of us went to the mall once because I needed a sweater. In spite of finding what I wanted in the first store we went to, we spent two hours in that mall. Every time Nelson spotted a child, he had to stop and ask the parents if there was anything he could do to help.

Finally John and I admitted that Nelson's mental condition had deteriorated. Even before his retirement he had told a story about himself—how he had circled twelve noon on his calendar one Friday and written the word "lunch" next to it. But then he couldn't remember with whom he was supposed to have lunch. Although he joked about the incident, it clearly bothered him—he had inconvenienced somebody, and he hated that.

"If Dad is as bad as I think he is, what would you say about my parents moving in with us?" John asked me.

I kissed him and told him I'd say yes.

With his mother's financial help, John and I bought twenty acres in the remote, high-desert area of Los Angeles County, since all of us prefer country to city life. Our plan was to build two houses, one on each ten-acre parcel and then move out of our small home in Pasadena. When we ran into opposition from the County Planning Commission, we temporarily leased a large enough home for all of us in Santa Clarita.

Moving was a nightmare for John's mother. Since she's a musician, they had an organ and a baby grand piano, in addition to all the usual furniture. Packing was the worst. Nelson questioned every item she put into every box. Several times he unpacked and hid things she had painstakingly packed the day before. But, when moving day arrived, she thought she was ready.

Nelson wasn't. As the movers struggled to carry a sofa to the truck he asked bitterly, "How can they get away with that? I worked hard all my life and here they are, stealing it all!" The movers returned for the baby grand. "Look at 'em," Nelson told John's mother. "A bunch of vultures—now wait just a minute there, young fella. That's heavier than it looks. Let me help you."

As soon as he laid a hand on the piano, the movers let go. Nelson wasn't an employee. If he got hurt "helping" them, they weren't willing to risk a lawsuit. All they could do was wait until John's mother lured Nelson out of the room to help her. A move that should have taken several hours ended up taking two days. Nelson's desire to help people was still stronger than his disease.

Once we were all together, the first thing we did was to establish some ground rules. John's parents would fix their own breakfast and lunch, and I would cook dinner for all of us. True to form, Nelson kept trying to "help." By then John and I had been to enough support group meetings to know that the best thing was to let Nelson help. While I made dinner, John and his parents usually sat in the family room to watch the news. The second I opened a drawer; Nelson would climb to his feet, come into the kitchen, and ask what he could do to help. I would give him some task—put placemats on the table or set out napkins. Once he had finished, he would sit back down in the family room. Two minutes later he would be back in the kitchen, asking me the same question.

We were all adjusting very well to a difficult situation, I thought, except that my hair rebelled. My hair is very straight and fine, and it did not like the desert air. It was getting dryer and more brittle with every breath I took. In addition, when I'm stressed, it starts falling out.

So, one afternoon, I walked into a "no appointment needed" shop and had most of it whacked off. When I returned home, John told me I looked like Tom Sawyer.

Our neighbors across the street happened to drop by that same afternoon to introduce themselves. When they asked what I did, I told them I taught at Antelope Valley College. "What do you teach?" the wife asked. "Physical education?"

With as much dignity as I could muster, I corrected her. "I'm an English teacher."

It's a practical haircut, I told myself. I'll wear it through the summer and then I'll figure out something else.

But that night, Nelson didn't come into the kitchen when I started banging pots around. Instead, after eyeing me for a few minutes from the family room, he turned to John's mother. "I'm hungry," he said. "When is that guy going to get out of the kitchen so Joan can cook?"

JOAN FRY

Making Sense of Time

On July 2, 2000, just one month before my father's ninetieth birthday, I jotted down the following notes from a conversation I had with my husband, David, and my father, Martin, at the nursing home where Martin lived.

Martin: "What time is it?"

Brenda: "11:40."

My father doesn't say a word but looks at me strangely.

David takes off his watch to show my father.

My father tilts his head to focus on David's watch.

David confirms the time: "See, it's 11:40!"

Martin: "Looks good enough to eat ... and then pass through and get rid of."

David tries to have fun with my father, and puts the watch in his mouth. Pulling it out, he asks, "Why would I want to eat my watch?"

Martin inquires, "When?"

BRENDA AVADIAN, MA
The Caregiver's Voice

Don't Eat the Yellow and Green Ones

This was our first and will probably be the last road trip with my little mama, who has Alzheimer's.

Although she kept saying she had a wonderful time, it was harder on her than I had expected. Being away from the safety and familiarity of our home made her more confused and she clung to me like a shadow. I tried to make things as easy as possible, to let her experience as much as she was able. To be honest, I think it was just as hard on me! But I really do think she enjoyed it. She's a real trooper!

First, we walked the beaches and collected shells along the coast.

Next, we spent the night at a place up in the mountains. There we saw seven deer (two mamas, two sets of twin babies, and one yearling). I witnessed the gleam of a child's joy on Mama's face as the babies romped in the grass; and then as the tired babies lay next to their mamas while being lovingly cleaned.

Actually, I got to see that childlike smile every place we took her. It was so precious!

We drove through the California desert. Even though we thought there was no beauty there, we came across a few flowers when we stopped to stretch our legs. Mama couldn't believe flowers grew in the desert. We now have one flower pressed between the pages of Mama's old family Bible.

We took her to places she had been before but she didn't remember them. It didn't matter, as long as she enjoyed it. (And I think she did!) Everything was new and an adventure for her, and we were able to share these experiences. The old memories are gone, but I am so thankful I had the chance to make new ones with her. I will hang onto these memories as Alzheimer's takes her further away.

After returning from our trip and getting everyone back into their routines (ruts!), I started writing some of the events in my quiet time—things we saw, things we shared and some of the silly little things we experienced on our "August 2000 Road Trip." I thought you might get a kick out of this part. <Grin>

During our vacation we either stayed at a motel or with family and friends. Three of us, Larry, Mama, and me, in one motel room—what a combination! I am glad I took my earplugs along!

Before we left, I looked around the house for the Ziploc® bag of earplugs I had collected over the years There were yellow, lime-green, white, and even a few orange pairs—all pretty, bright colors. I figured I wouldn't need them all but what the heck; I threw the whole bag in the suitcase since they didn't take any room.

On the nights when Larry and my little mama snored so loud they raised the roof clean off the whole building, not even earplugs helped!!! Have you ever heard snoring in stereo? <Grin> I'm surprised they didn't charge us extra for the room!

In the evenings, before we turned off the lights, I'd get out those earplugs, get "plugged," and leave the bag sitting on the nightstand between the two beds. Hmmmm, that was not a good plan!

The first morning, as we were waking up, my little mama sat on the side of the bed, grabbed the bag full of earplugs, and reached in. "What ya' doing?" I asked.

Like a child caught with her hand in the bag, she asked, "What? Can't I have some of this candy?"

As she pulled out one of the earplugs from the bag, I hollered, "NOOOOOOOOOO, those are MY EARPLUGS!"

We all cracked up, as she quickly put the bag back on the nightstand and said, "Oh, I thought they were marshmallows!!!"

What more could I ask for then to start the day with a smile? Three mornings in a row, no matter where I put the Ziploc® bag, she found it. I always caught her just before she put the earplugs in her mouth. Mama couldn't remember from the day before what they were, so we would have to explain it all again.

I was afraid that one of these mornings I would be awakened by my little mama plucking "marshmallows" out of my ears!

The fourth morning I thought I had hidden them pretty well. She hadn't been rummaging through our suitcases (or so I thought) and figured they would be safe. But, nooooooooo ... Larry woke me just as she was lifting the lid to my suitcase, and guess what she found? You got it! MARSHMALLOWS! So I motioned to Larry to be still and we lay quietly and watched as she popped a couple in her mouth. We tried our best not to laugh out loud as Mama walked as fast as her little feet could move to the sink to SPIT them OUT!!!!

Now, I know it sounds mean, but though I tried in every way to tell her they weren't candy, she had it in her mind to get a taste of those marshmallows. No one was going to change her mind! This time we just didn't stop her from getting that taste!!!

Thank goodness we didn't have a problem the rest of the trip. I guess they weren't as sweet as she thought they would be! I thought, "FINALLY, the message got through to her! Problem solved!"

HA!

After we came home, I unpacked and left some things on the dining room table. Of course, one of those things was the Ziploc® bag of earplugs! I walked in the back door with my hands full of pillows, empty Pepsi® cans, and more. Lo and behold, there was my little mama, sitting in her rocking chair, about to eat a few "marshmallows," AGAIN!

Now, I have one question for you. How is it that she can forget EVERYTHING else but I couldn't get her to forget those earplugs?

LORAINE YATES (WILLO)

(Author's Note: After meeting online, Loraine and I met in person. We continue to forge a wonderful relationship. I consider her a member of my caregiving family. With her permission I have included this slightly edited version of her e-mail to me.)

"Who's the father?"

On Father's Day in 1998, I visited my father in the nursing home to celebrate his special day. Except we couldn't agree on whose special day it really was!

"Oh, I'm glad you're here!" he said with a bright smile.

His eyes told the truth. He no longer remembered his daughter with whom he shared a birthday.

He looked right at me. I could have been the nurse's assistant or an aide. Sometimes I was his son.

"Happy Father's Day!" I said, with as much enthusiasm as I could muster.

"Father's Day?" he asked. "Who's the father?"

"You are!" I said, hoping he would remember.

"I am?" he asked, pointing awkwardly at himself. He paused, and then shaking his head, retorted, "You're the father!"

BRENDA AVADIAN, MA
The Caregiver's Voice

Whose Prosthesis is This Anyway?

About twenty years ago, my mom had a radical mastectomy of her left breast. She wears a gel prosthesis. At night before going to bed, she removes it and puts it in the drawer. She spends about ten minutes every morning looking for it because she forgets where she puts it. She never forgets that she has a prosthesis.

Many times, when I help her get dressed, especially while pulling her sweatshirt over her head and down her chest, her prosthesis slips down and falls to the floor. We both laugh because she makes a funny comment in Spanish, "Cuidado, no seáis tan tosco. No mas me queda una mas." ("Careful, don't be so rough. I only have one left.")

After twenty years, it began to leak and the gel inside ran all over her chest. It was time to get Mom a new prosthesis.

While the new one was on order, she tried a temporary one made of foam rubber. It was shaped exactly like a breast, and even had a nipple. However, my mom did not recognize it as her normal prosthesis, so she was reluctant to use it.

One Sunday morning we were getting ready to go out for breakfast. I heard her going through her dresser drawers. After a while, I asked her what she was looking for.

Flustered, she said she was trying to find her prosthesis so she could get ready.

I found the temporary prosthesis and asked her to put it on.

She looked at it and said, "Eso no es mio." ("That is not mine.")

I reminded her that it was a temporary one, until her permanent one arrived. I told her to put it on while I wait for her in the kitchen.

She came out a few minutes later and was ready to go.

At the restaurant, my mom's nose was running a little and I asked her to get some tissues from her purse. At that moment a waitress came to the table to take our order. As I was giving the waitress our order, my mom was pulling items out of her purse and placing them on the table. Suddenly, the waitress' face contorted into an expression of total shock and amazement.

I looked at my mom, her purse, and then looked at the table. One of the items my mother had removed from her purse and placed on the table was the foam-rubber prosthesis. She continued looking for a tissue.

I quickly hid the prosthesis and continued to give the waitress our order. My mom was completely unaware of what she had done.

I will never forget the look on the waitress' face.

When the waitress left with our order, I asked my mother to put her prosthesis back in her purse.

She looked at me and exclaimed, "Eso no es mio!"

I quickly tucked it away in my jacket to avoid further incident. Now, I looked like I was missing a breast!

GIL LOZANO
Retired Engineer

SECTION II

Children Show the Way

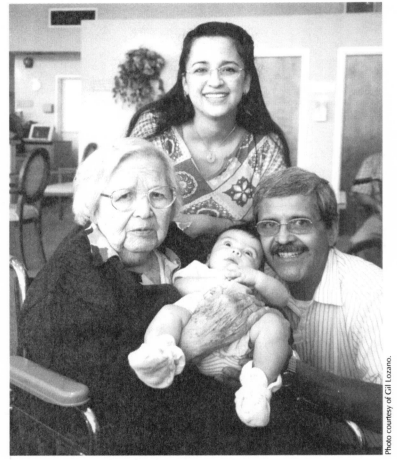

Four generations of the Lozano family.
Stories from Gil Lozano (seated on the right) appear in this book.

Many caregivers who shared their stories are adult children writing about their parents. Their stories, especially those that involve young children, teach us so much because children, by virtue of their youth and innocence, tend to capture the essence of life. Children enthusiastically embrace the hope that comes with living. Their stories are found throughout this book.

A few of these stories appear in this section. Whether it is ten-year-old Caleb Stephen Jordan turning "Good Things Out of Bad," as his grandmother struggles with Alzheimer's disease or Ricky teaching his mother, Mandy, an important lesson in Mary Emma Allen's touching story "A Child Shows the Way."

On the other hand, adult children are often thrust into a role reversal with their parents. Awkward at first, the adult child—turned caregiver—must learn to protect the parent from danger and to be firm when necessary. As funny as the circumstances may be, this is one of the hardest things for caregivers to accept, as in "When Our Parents Become Our Children."

Caregivers found abundant joys, some as simple as "Saving a Life with Breakfast." I fondly recall a bittersweet moment when my father wanted to die, then changed his mind once breakfast was ready.

A Child Shows the Way

"I'm here, Granny," Ricky announced.

Mandy watched the small boy touch the old lady's hand and smile at her.

Mom Perkins looked blankly at him and said nothing.

Ricky didn't seem to care. He kept chattering away. "Can we take Granny for a ride to see the lights, Mama?" he asked.

Mandy wondered what was the use. Her mother wouldn't know whether there were Christmas lights or not. She didn't realize it was Christmas, the season she always enjoyed.

They wheeled Mom Perkins into the activity room. There, the nursing home's Christmas tree shone with twinkling lights and carols peeled forth from a CD player.

"See the lights, Granny?" asked Ricky, pointing to the colored lights. "And here's a Christmas ball. It has a picture of baby Jesus in the manger."

Mom Perkins didn't respond. But Ricky kept talking.

"She doesn't understand!" Mandy felt like shouting to her son. She's not the person I remember, Mandy thought as she recalled childhood Christmas celebrations when her mother played a prominent role.

Then Ricky tugged at her arm.

"Granny smiled at me, Mama," he said with a grin. "She likes the lights."

Oh, yeah, thought Mandy.

Ricky continued, "See, she's moving her hand to the music."

Yes, Mom Perkins was patting the arm of the wheelchair, almost as though she heard the music.

"She always liked Christmas carols," Mandy explained to Ricky. "She liked to take us to church on Christmas when we sang carols."

"She still likes them, Mama," said Ricky.

Then he began patting the arm of the chair along with his grandmother.

This is what Christmas is all about, thought Mandy, beginning to feel more at peace. A smile came to her face as she watched her son and mother. Ricky has shown me how to enjoy someone even when they can't respond or be the person we remember. I have to accept Mom where she is.

Mandy realized, too, that her mother could still enjoy Christmas, but at a different level now.

It took a little boy to show me, she thought.

"Let's take her to see more Christmas decorations, Mama," said Ricky.

Mandy helped Ricky push Mom Perkins down the hall to see a Christmas wreath with a bright red and silver bow.

Before they left the nursing home, Ricky placed an ornament he'd made on the nightstand beside the bed ... a gift for his Granny.

But his greater gift is accepting her where she's at, thought Mandy, and teaching me to do the same.

MARY EMMA ALLEN
Author and Speaker

(Editor's note: This story first appeared in The Ribbon *in the winter of 2000.)*

Good Things Out of Bad

My grandmother has Alzheimer's. It has been very sad for everyone that knows her. But along with the sadness of Alzheimer's have come happy moments—times when my mom, our whole family, and me have been able to laugh.

I call my grandmother "Nana." Ever since my mom and I moved Nana up to Grand Junction, Colorado from Dallas, Texas, we have seen a serious decrease in my grandmother's memory. My new step-dad, Tim Frasier, and his kids, Travis (19), Savanah (16), Spencer (13), and Lance (10, about a half-year younger than me) also noticed a difference. But we have all been able to laugh.

Some people might say that our laughing is rude, but we look at it as pretending someone is a very good comedian (my grandmother), even though she might not laugh herself.

One thing that we laugh about is Nana's passing fads. About six months ago, she began, and continues today, to look up at the sky and say, "Looks like it's gonna rain," even if there is not a cloud in the sky. Other times, wherever there is grass, she will exclaim, "That grass sure is green!" She says this even if the grass is dead. She also looks at every tree and says, "I'll bet that's a peach tree." She says these phrases over and over. About a month ago, she started mimicking my mom, but changing everything slightly so that everyone would start cracking up silently.

Some of her actions can be funny, too. One time, when my mom and I were moving Nana from her room in our house to Nana's house next door, Mom asked Nana to carry a box to her house. Nana picked it up, carried it to the garage, and then returned carrying the box back to our house. We laughed.

Nana has come up with nicknames for my cat, Aspen, because she can't remember his name. Aspen is known for tearing through the house and knocking chairs over at ninety miles per hour. Here are some of Nana's nicknames for Aspen: Skidso, Speedo, and Psycho.

All these funny things just go to show that Alzheimer's can help people make the best of life. Alzheimer's could even be a fable with the moral, "Make the best of a bad situation."

CALEB STEPHEN JORDAN
Age: 10

When Our Parents Become Our Children

What if you became your parent's parent? What would it be like to be your *mother's* parent? What would you do if your *father* tried to shoplift?

In September 1996, my husband, David, and I moved my father from his Wisconsin home of forty-five years into our southern California home. A few months after the move my eighty-seven-year-old father and I were shopping at a local department store. He spotted a wallet misplaced in the candy aisle. "Hey, a wallet! I'll look at it later," he said, as he discreetly placed it in his pocket.

I smiled and thought he was being cute. But he refused to put it back. I feared he might be arrested, handcuffed, and taken to jail for shoplifting.

Then I imagined him in a panic, wondering what had happened and why people were restraining him. I would be helpless once the law stepped in. My father, a man who had never committed a crime, would be traumatized. He wouldn't understand why he was in jail.

Anticipating these consequences, I asked, "Mardig (We called him by his first name, Mardig, which is Armenian for Martin.), is that yours?"

"Shoosh," he said sternly, placing his index finger to his lips.

I grew more serious, "No, Mardig. Is that wallet yours?"

"Well, it's not theirs!" he exclaimed. "Because if it was, they would know where to place it," he reasoned.

I was perplexed. How do I get an adult, *my father*, to listen to me? "Please, Mardig. Take that wallet out of your pocket, now!" I insisted firmly in a low tone of voice. I didn't want to get him riled up.

"No!" he exclaimed and began to walk ahead of me.

"Mardig," I caught up to him and pulled his left arm as his hand gripped the wallet in his pocket. "Please, you must give me that wallet. You can get arrested for stealing. You could go to jail!"

"Well, no one will know about it if you keep your voice down," he said sternly.

Finally, I pulled his arm out of his pocket and reached into his left pocket and removed the wallet—to his loud objections.

As I stood in that department store, irritated at my father's behavior, I feared what others might perceive as a younger adult accosting an older man and stealing his wallet.

Yet, just as a responsible parent ensures that his/her child follows the rules, I too had to make sure that my father followed the law. The only difference was that a parent can teach his/her child what is right. And, over time, the child will *learn*. My *child*, my father, could no longer learn because Alzheimer's disease was destroying his brain. This terminal disease—his death sentence—was taking my father away, piece-by-piece, from those he loved and from those who loved him.

My father and I share a birthday—August 22. I came into this world on his forty-ninth. Throughout my life, we were known as "the two Leos." My father would always say, "We Leos have to stick together."

Up until age ninety, when my father passed away, he needed help with the basic functions of life that many of us take for granted—toileting, dressing, showering, and even eating. He no longer recognized his *fellow Leo.*

My father lived in a skilled nursing facility. Although he did not know me, I visited him a couple of hours once or twice a week. I helped feed him and accepted what the disease allowed us to share during the time we had together.

The bittersweet joys are what caregivers learn to accept. As we slowly lose our loved ones the joys get simpler and smaller, like feeding my father his dinner.

BRENDA AVADIAN, MA
The Caregiver's Voice

(Editor's Note: The preceding is adapted from an article the author wrote, which has found its way into fifteen countries.)

Saving a Life with Breakfast

About three months after we moved my father from his Wisconsin home into our California home, he appeared to be troubled by something.

He was usually up and wandering early; trying to find his shoes so he could leave for work. He must have been up during the night because when I walked into his bedroom that morning to invite him to breakfast, he was sleeping in his rocking chair.

I decided to return later, when breakfast was ready.

When I came back, he was waking from his slumber.

"Good morning, Mardig!" I greeted him with a big smile.

"Good morning," he said.

"Whatcha doing?" I asked playfully.

He paused, his eyes glimmering with hope, and asked, "Are you busy?"

"No," I replied, curious about the look on his face.

"Come in here then," he said, "and sit down." He motioned toward the rocking chair.

I hesitated because I didn't want the food to get cold. But he quickly stood up to close the door and said, "I don't want him to hear," referring to my husband, David.

Thinking this was one of those moments when he shared a secret with either David or me, I decided to indulge him for a minute or two and sat on the spare chair in his room.

He sat on the rocking chair that had been in our family since I was a child. His voice softened and he looked down and slightly away, "I want your advice."

"Yes?" I inquired, concerned for him and the seriousness in his voice.

"Do you know of anyone who ... who ... a doctor who can prescribe pills ... I don't want you to get into any trouble."

"What do you need, Mardig?" I asked gently, knowing he was feeling funny about something.

He motioned for me to lean close, "I don't want him to hear ... *I want to die.*" He articulated each of the four words to make sure I heard.

My heart skipped a few beats and I gulped to catch my breath. I knew this was difficult for him to say. I tried to help him feel comfortable. "So, you want to die, Mardig?"

"Yes!" he said, with a sense of relief.

I tried not to show my surprise. I wanted him to feel his request was normal. Yet, I needed to know. "Why?" I asked.

"Because there's nothing to do around here."

"What do you mean, Mardig? You've got a lot of reading to do!" I said, directing his attention to the filled bookshelves behind him.

He made a half-hearted attempt to turn and look at them and then turned back. "I forget things. I can't find the words to say what I mean. Do you know that?"

"You seem to do fine for me," I said to reassure and comfort him.

"I do?" he asked, surprised.

"Yes, I enjoy our conversations," I added.

"Conversations, monversations," he belittled the importance. "A man can't live by conversation alone. A man has to work."

"Look," he said, serious again. "Do you know of any doctor who can help give me something … or do something, so it doesn't get back to you and you don't get into any trouble … I don't want you to get into any trouble … to help me die?"

"Kevorkian," I blurted out.

"Huh?" he asked.

"Oh, nothing," I said. I didn't know why I said that.

"Well, I suppose there are things, but you must realize it is illegal to try and take your own life. What if you don't succeed and live as a vegetable?" I tried to appeal to his rational side.

"Oh," he said thoughtfully. Then he took a deep breath, sat up straight, and said, "Hey, you came in here! I don't want to take your time. What are you doing?"

"Making breakfast for us," I said.

He smiled and replied, "Oh, okay … is it ready?"

"Yes," I said.

He placed both hands on the arms of the rocker, hoisted himself up, and eagerly followed me to the dining room.

BRENDA AVADIAN, MA
The Caregiver's Voice

SECTION III

Loving Couples

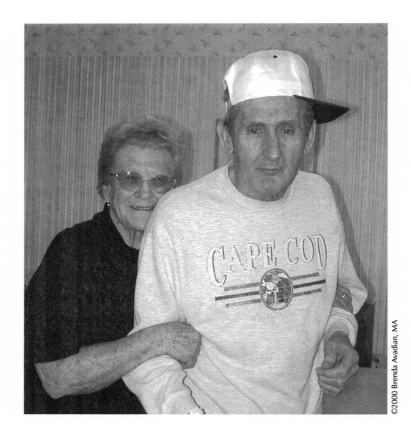

Marion and Don Riley.

Spouses, life-long partners, and lovers facing this disease share joyful moments—despite the terminal sentence they have been given. Each faces the realization that Alzheimer's will take one of them away. Imagine spending your life with someone, growing to love that person, to feel comfortable and secure with him or her, only to know that you will live the rest of your life without that person. How do you go on? Evelyn Daniel put pen to paper and wrote a bittersweet poem, "Dreams Swept In."

You and your partner may have been together twenty, forty, or even fifty years. One couple I know has been married for sixty-six years! The husband has Alzheimer's and lives in the skilled nursing facility that my father lived in. His loving wife is eighty-nine years young and visits him nearly every day.

As the years add up, these couples' lives become a multi-textured fabric called LIFE from which we, in the generations that follow, can learn so much.

As we face the prospect of losing a partner, how do we cope with the need for companionship, for intimacy, and for a balanced and socialized life? " 'Do you take … in sickness and in health?' 'I do.' " by Sharon DeMoe gives us one perspective. How do we take on the additional responsibilities that our partner can no longer fulfill? " 'May I help you?' " is the story of how one World War II veteran still finds joy, even though he is losing his "teammate."

Spouses are in a unique caregiving situation. They have no one to go home to, to confide in. If their partner is in a nursing home, the well partner goes home to an empty house. They have no one to share dinner with or to discuss and share opinions. Alone, they must carry out their lives. The nature of their love changes toward compassion borne out of caregiving, and even sadness, for their spouses. Jonathan Schulkin writes about his wife of sixty years, whose speech was undecipherable until one day ... in "Those Three Words."

Contrary to popular perceptions, many caregivers continue to lead active and involved lives. Some volunteer, sometimes working harder than they did during their careers. Others go to social events—dinners, dances, and even pre-arranged tours to exotic places. I am impressed with the increasing numbers who actively use computers and are on the Internet. And they are in their eighties! The saying: "Old dogs can't learn new tricks" hardly applies to these active folks. Some, at twice my age, can still teach me a thing or two!

Finally, Rosa Lee Boslar's "Sonny Sagas" is the hardship-to-JOY story that gives caregivers hope in the face of difficult circumstances and leaves the reader with the feeling that a life-changing decision was the right one.

Dreams Swept In

My heart had stifled every thought of you
And all the lovely dreams you left to me
I swept in heaps to be forgotten, too
It is a most distressing sight to see
A Heart so locked and sealed against the world
Fearing the name, the voice of one grown dear.

I had not thought that I, securely curled
Within your ardent arms, would ever fear
The dreadfulness, the bleakness of despair
A life without you full of sounds and sights
So fraught with memr'y that I could not bear
The bitter empty days and barren nights.

I swept all the dreams out of my heart and then—
Then, I remembered you and swept them in again.

EVELYN DANIEL

"Do you take ... in sickness and in health?"
"I do."

Are there joyful moments in my life? Do I experience joy while I care for my fifty-four-year-old husband who has early-onset Alzheimer's disease? Absolutely!

My husband was diagnosed six years ago. Soon after, he began losing his ability to communicate. This loss is typical for people with Alzheimer's, although some are able to communicate for a longer time than others. My husband's difficulty communicating frequently presents a problem. I have to explain and repeat things to him. I assume he is also losing his ability to comprehend as he approaches the middle stage of this disease. Despite this, there is a bright side. Having lived with him for thirty-two years, I have become quite skilled at guessing and mind reading.

As other caregivers have shared with me, there are good days and bad days. A good day is usually when nothing unusual or stressful happens. A bad day is when several things happen. He may do something completely unexpected or behave in a way that is dangerous. Once, he tried to get out of our car while we were going down the highway at sixty-five miles per hour. Luckily he didn't succeed, but I started looking into child safety locks for our car.

Do I "lose it?" Yes, more often than I care to admit. I lose my patience, raise my voice, get angry with him, and, sometimes I cry in front of him. After much prayer, God gives me the ability to find joy and humor in these situations.

On our wedding day, thirty-two years ago, we each made promises to God and to each other. We promised that we would love each other in sickness and in health, for better or worse, and for richer or poorer, until death do us part. These promises we made brought me comfort and joy, because we became at that moment, not two separate people just getting married. We became one, together for eternity.

I know in my heart that if the tables were turned and I was ill, my husband would be by my side, loving me, and caring for me. Possibly he would be doing a better job than I am doing. And that has brought me tremendous security and joy.

Those who know us say my husband is easy to love. I agree. He is a wonderful husband, father, and grandfather. We continually find happiness in our marriage. It is not as it was before, but we do have our special moments. There are times when we hear an old 50's song we like, and we jump up and dance a few minutes together. Or, during the day, when we're casually passing each other, we'll give each other a little pat or a tickle. And there are the little smiles and hugs we share when the words are just too hard to verbalize.

My husband has always been fun loving. Occasionally, he will intentionally do something funny. Or, there are times when he thinks I am being funny. Then something wonderful happens—we laugh so hard together that we end up crying big, soggy, joyful tears.

I admit that my retirement isn't what I dreamed it would be. But all the wonderful memories of yesteryear and those we make together now will help us through our struggles with this disease.

There are other things that bring me happiness, which don't involve my husband. They bring some balance into my life. I enjoy shopping with my daughters and friends, as I believe every red-blooded American woman does, and I personally believe that God never intended for a husband and wife to be together twenty-four hours a day, seven days a week.

I also enjoy working jigsaw puzzles. I call this my "brainless" hobby, as it gives me an opportunity not to think about what is going on. And, the computer has given me access to a tremendous amount of information about Alzheimer's disease. In the process, I have gained many new and dear friends. These last two activities allow me to stay home and care for my husband.

Finally, I am delighted to spend time with our family. Our two daughters are the apples of my husband's eye, but my heart melts each time his eyes light up when he sees our granddaughters.

I understand the heartache and many challenges in the everyday life of a caregiver. It seems as though we are on a roller coaster ride most of the time. In my heart, I believe I can survive this so-called abnormal life. I will care for my husband as long as I am mentally and physically able. Not only because I love him but also because in the midst of the confusion and turmoil there are heartfelt, humorous, and revitalizing moments of joy in my life.

SHARON DeMoE

"May I help you?"

After serving four years in the Army Air Corps during World War II, I joined the family business and became involved in community activities. I served on the board of the local Chamber of Commerce and participated in the Air Corps reserve training program. My wife became active in community organizations as well, among them the United Crusade and the Girl Scout Council, where she served as president.

We've been married fifty-five years and have three wonderful daughters and seven beautiful grandchildren. During these years, we actively participated in community groups and organizations.

"Teamwork" has been our byword. If one needed help with a project the other was always ready to assist. This made our efforts so much more enjoyable.

However, teamwork has been somewhat of a challenge lately. My wife was diagnosed with Alzheimer's disease and she cannot always handle the chores. This has frustrated her, since she is well aware of what is happening. She berates herself for her inability to function as she did before. Guilt prods her for her inability to perform.

To counter this, she has become obsessed with the idea of helping me. She is constantly asking if there is something she can do, something to help me with—whatever I am doing.

Much of my effort now is devoted to paperwork; taking care of our investments and following up on correspondence.

She pops into my office constantly, asking what she can do to help. She reminds me that she loves me, and wants to be of assistance, if at all possible.

I tell her how much I love her and how appreciative I am of her willingness to help me.

Occasionally there is a chore that she can handle, and doing it gives her such a lift. What a thrill for her to prove herself, that she is not completely washed up!

This is one of the small joys of caring for my wife as this disease gradually takes my teammate from me—to see her being so considerate and willing to help whenever she can.

A. Nony Mous

Sonny Sagas

My husband, Sonny, worked for General Telephone for forty-four years. Each time new telephone equipment came onto the market he went to school to be certified. He was a smart man and learned quickly. He could easily fix things, including computers, household items, and our car.

When Sonny turned sixty-five he retired. We bought a new motorhome so that we could travel. Our first trip was to Seattle, Washington. Before we left on this trip, I had noticed that Sonny was forgetting things. I figured he was just getting older. But during our trip to Seattle, he had difficulty reading the map or remembering the directions I gave. Several times he'd ask me to repeat the directions. This became very frustrating for both of us.

When we got home, I told our children that I thought something was terribly wrong with their father.

Shortly after, Sonny was diagnosed with prostate cancer. While he was in the hospital, I actually thought he had had a stroke because he was acting so strange. The doctor told me it was the pain medication Sonny was taking.

I took him to the doctor for several follow-up visits after the surgery. During Sonny's routine physical, I told the doctor I thought something was wrong. She said that when people get older they become forgetful and suggested that I have patience, despite my continued concern. Meanwhile, Sonny was saying he was just fine and that I was the one who had the problem.

After several more months, Sonny started to have difficulty fixing things around the house. He couldn't handle the checkbook or even go to the grocery store to buy milk or bread. (Sonny had always done the marketing, banking, and fixing of things that needed repair.)

Many more months passed and I noticed things getting worse. Sonny was losing his short-term memory. He couldn't remember what we had just talked about, or that I had asked him to take out the trash. Not satisfied with the doctor's responses to my concerns I insisted that she refer Sonny to a neurologist.

He was diagnosed with Alzheimer's.

During the months that followed, I tended to Sonny's every need. I was exhausted. He would pace the floor and leave the house. I was losing my patience and screamed at him to sit down and stay put. I got so tired of following him up and down the hallway in our home, or running outside to bring him back into the house.

Sonny could no longer bathe, shave, or dress himself. Things got complicated when he forgot where the bathroom was. I even had to tie him to me at night so I would know when he got out of bed. I got up with him two and three times at night just to help him use the bathroom. Cleaning up after him and always trying to be one step ahead of his needs became too much for one person twenty-four hours a day.

Despite my exhaustion, it was hard for me to place Sonny in a nursing home. I knew they had a full-time staff to take care of Sonny around the clock. I remember the unexpected relief and joy I felt when I dropped him off the first day. But this sense of relief was quickly followed by shame and guilt; to think I could just abandon my husband so easily. How could I have done such a thing, just because I was too tired to go on taking care of him?

I began attending the caregiver support group meetings at the nursing home. I soon found out that my feelings were normal, and that most caregivers felt the same, whether placing their spouse or parent. I began to accept that this was the best thing I could have done for my husband.

Sonny has been in a nursing home for two years now. I have finally been able to regain some balance in my life. I am still limited to what I am able to do because I am actively involved in Sonny's care. Sonny has become a child (again) in an adult body, with every care and need being tended to by the staff at the nursing home. But the respite from having to care for him twenty-four hours a day has helped me to enjoy the time I spend with him.

I can now look beyond Sonny and find humor in some of the things that go on where he lives.

In the nursing home is a man who is small in stature, gentle, and has a wonderful smile. Sometimes he is a little flirtatious. One day, as I walked toward the facility to visit Sonny, I noticed how the sun shined brightly on one of the windows. And then I clearly saw this man sitting in a chair sunning himself. The only thing was, he was naked! When he saw me, his face brightened with a sheepishly naughty, flirtatious grin, as if to say, "Look at me, and I don't even care!" I smiled and waved to him and proceeded into the facility.

On another occasion, I was sitting in the multipurpose room, where the residents can get snacks and coffee, listen to music, play games, and, those who cannot feed themselves, get help with their meals. As I sat beside my husband, a female resident approached Sonny and asked him for two bucks. When my husband just sat there staring at her, she asked again and said she needed to buy cat food. When Sonny did not reply the second time, she turned to me and asked, "What's the matter with him?"

Another time I went to visit, I found my husband strolling down the hall holding hands with a female resident. I told her she would have to let go of his hand because he had to go with me.

She asked, "Who are you?"

"I am his wife," I replied.

She inquired in a huff, "His wife? You mean I've been living with him all this time and he never told me he was married!"

❦   ❦   ❦

Every day, I try to find something to laugh about, or I'll spend my days crying.

ROSA LEE BOSLAR

Those Three Words

I am convinced that most caregivers of people with Alzheimer's, particularly those in the advanced stages of the disease, find little cause for jubilation in the experience. Yet there are times when a ray of light shines through the darkness.

My wife, Elizabeth, has been in the grip of Alzheimer's for nearly ten years—five years at home and almost five years in a nursing facility. In all these years she has accepted her situation with remarkable equanimity, despite occasional damaging falls and infections. Although I visit her consistently and she seems to know who I am, it has been frustrating to me to hear her talk but not be able to decipher what she is saying because the words don't come out right.

But one recent day at lunchtime, as I was feeding her, she suddenly said, loud and clear, "I love you." The amazement of the nurse's aides, who also heard it, confirmed that I had not imagined it. Well, that made my day for a week! And the same "miracle" occurred the following week, when she uttered the same three little words.

It gladdens my heart to know that after sixty years of married life there still exists this bond between us.

JONATHAN SCHULKIN

SECTION IV

Friends are Like Family

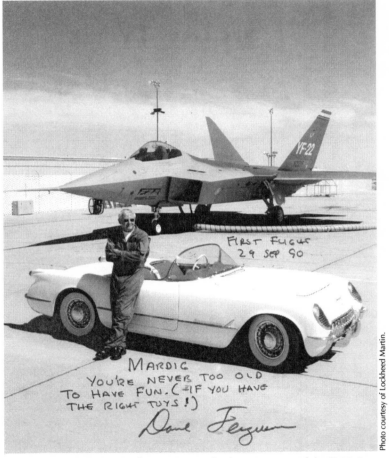

Handwriting on photo:

FIRST FLIGHT
29 SEP 90

MARDIC
YOU'RE NEVER TOO OLD
TO HAVE FUN. (#IF YOU HAVE
THE RIGHT TOYS!)

Dave Ferguson

Dave ("Ferg") Ferguson, first person to fly the prototype of the F-22 (in the background), standing by his other toy—a '53 Corvette. Ferg and his wife, Jan, helped care for Martin Avadian.

Friends are the special people in our lives we think of when we want to celebrate an occasion or when we need help. They often fill in when family cannot. With families moving farther apart and careers taking us to different cities, or even countries, we have a greater need to feel a sense of community, bonding, or "family." Friends often fill this void.

Those who are able to reach out to friends will find many pleasures.

Several years ago, I chose to stay home to be near my father for the Easter holiday, even though I felt a little sad about missing David's family's Easter celebration. Instead, David and I decided to celebrate Easter at our home and to invite my other "family"—caregivers in our support group. Some had also found themselves in the same situation, having decided to stay home to be near their loved ones.

Since we had only known each other for two or three years (in the support group) we didn't share any of the history that sometimes makes family gatherings stressful. We truly enjoyed one another's company. Everything we learned about each other was new. We laughed, we ate, we talked, and we drank. We really had a GREAT time! It actually turned out so well we continue the tradition for different occasions, such as birthdays, holidays, and anniversaries.

Friends are near to cheer us on when we achieve our goal. They're by our side when we are sad and struggling. Their perspectives give us something to consider when we are burdened with the day-to-day challenges of caring for our loved ones.

Sometimes they'll do more to help. In *"Where's my shoes?" My Father's Walk Through Alzheimer's*, I wrote about two very special families—the Fergusons and the Howards. Both families heroically stepped in to help care for my father when I was out of town on business and while David faced thirteen-hour days away from home commuting and at work.

Since David and I don't have children, I used to wonder what we would do when we grew old. Would we be alone? Would anyone pay attention? Would anyone care? One of the important lessons I learned on this journey is that we will only be alone if we choose to be. With families spread far apart, it is hard for family members to get together. Besides, parents don't like to burden their children. So many are at risk of being alone in their older years. But this doesn't have to be. In "A Prayer Answered," Mary Barrass writes an inspiring story of how she gained a friend and family member despite the many losses and heartbreaks she suffered.

Each of us wants to have an impact in the world. Sometimes the one who carries on our legacy is a friend we barely know. "Family of Friends" is the story about a woman whose legacy lives on through those whose lives she's touched. One, in particular, has taken a tremendous step toward helping others in her honor. Often we have had an impact and we don't really give it much thought, until years later when someone unexpected comes forth to help us. And sometimes this comes from a family member who acts as a dear friend. "Is it C.R.S. or Alzheimer's?" is the story of how Eula Youngblood became actively involved in her sister's care when her sister's husband and children did not.

Finally, "David's Pink Purse" emphasizes the camaraderie shared among friends when one's struggle to remember due to vascular dementia is met with the kind of love and support you might expect from family members.

Family of Friends

I dedicate this story to the loving memory of a dear online friend, "AlzJane198"—Jane Levy. Jane passed away on Valentine's Day 1999. Through the lives she touched via the Internet, Jane still continues to inspire, teach, and show compassion to caregivers struggling to care for their loved ones with Alzheimer's. Those who were graced by knowing Jane keep her deep in their hearts. Caregivers who did not meet her are still touched by her grace. She is our guardian angel.

I miss you, my friend. I know you are smiling at us now!

My father was diagnosed with Alzheimer's in early 1997. It hit all of us very hard, especially my mother. Even to this day, with my father living in a nursing home, my mom has not been able to come to grips with this disease. The eldest of two children, I moved from our home in the Midwest to California twenty years ago. My brother Ray remained in the area and has been a constant source of support for my mom.

Living nearly 2,000 miles away, I often have feelings of helplessness. At times, I drive myself crazy trying to second guess what my family is telling me. I can't return home often, and my family understands this.

It is said that out of something bad, something good will come. Alzheimer's has brought me many blessings.

Just before my father's diagnosis, my brother married. His wife, Teresa, became a wonderful addition to our family. She jumped right in and learned all she could. She even took the lead. With a new baby and twin boys, she helped my parents as much as she could. How fortunate we were that she came into our lives.

Of all things, the computer became my blessing. Through Internet chat rooms, online newsletters, etc., I was able to meet people and learn more about my father's disease. Despite the distance, I stay involved with my father's care by sharing what I learn with my family. As a long-distance caregiver, I've gained a second-hand perspective from primary caregivers online.

An unexpected gift presented itself to me one night when I stumbled into an Internet chat room filled with people from across the country. Here were caregivers going through the same problems my family was facing. Not being bashful, I jumped right in and began asking question after question.

During my initial visit I met Jane Levy. She lost her mother seventeen years earlier to Alzheimer's and was still helping people who needed support. As I came to know Jane, I regarded her as a precious jewel. She granted me one of the major joys during my long-distance caregiving journey. As often is the case with the Internet, I never met her personally and only spoke with her once on the telephone.

Yet, Jane still remains my inspiration. Her heart and compassion for people was steadfast. During those two brief years I got to know her well. We discussed the possibility of creating a website to assist caregivers. Sadly, she passed away shortly thereafter. She left a gaping void and was never able to see our vision come to fruition.

Because Jane's life had inspired and touched mine so deeply,

I decided to go forth with the website. Enlisting the support of a group of online friends, we began fitting the pieces of the puzzle together. Kevin, a young man of only fourteen years, designed the web page. Joyce, a dear friend in South Carolina, found the graphic for the page. It is a scene of a latticed porch. A book sits on a rocking chair, and an afghan drapes across the swing on the porch. A path leads from the houses in the background to this porch. It invites the caregiver, "Come, this is the place to relax, get cozy, and find friends who will accompany you on the road you have traveled alone." Meanwhile, Mary, a friend in Washington, kept after me to see the project through. After seven months of work and fine-tuning, the site opened. (You are invited to visit at http://www.theribbon/GatherPlace/.)

The Gathering Place has been a constant source of joy for me and for those who visit. It was a rough road, but the challenges made us relish the joy all the more. After a year at our original site, we were truly honored when our friends Jamie, Karen, and Kevin from *The Ribbon* (http://www. theribbon. com) invited us to join their team.

Wonderful friendships blossom at The Gathering Place. What a blessing. Caregivers come to The Gathering Place because they are lost, bewildered, or almost ready to give up. I'm amazed as the "old-timers" spring to life and pull these over-whelmed caregivers under their wings. I sit and smile. Other times I shed tears of joy when the experienced caregivers, who haven't quite dealt with their own pain, encourage a new person to share their situation. The greatest gift is watching the new caregivers learn to accept they are not on this journey alone, that there are warm, wonderful, and caring folks who have been down the path. I am crying with joy as I reflect on this.

While on vacation at my cousin Barbara's home, I invited her to The Gathering Place. She was astounded at how the folks tried to help a new caregiver. She told me she was proud of what we had accomplished, of the avenue The Gathering Place provided to caregivers, and of the many lives that have been touched and are yet to be touched.

What a truly joyous experience it was to finally meet several of my online friends face-to-face. I vowed, after not having met Jane, that I would try to meet some of these very special folks. I now have two new, wonderful "sisters," Mary and Sharon, and I've traveled around the country and met many more online friends—all who I consider special angels.

It is my hope that all who read this will take a slightly different view. It is a horrible, horrible disease; no one could ever argue that. Yet, I have found that those people I meet—face-to-face, through letters, via the telephone, or on the Internet—can have a positive impact on how I cope with this disease.

I believe that if one looks at caregiving openly and honestly, one will see what a blessing it is that a Higher Power saw the special qualities in a person to entrust him or her with a loved one's care.

To think, these are all the blessings I count after my father was diagnosed with Alzheimer's.

LINDA/PHOTOLJT
The Gathering Place, Online Alzheimer's Caregiver Support

A Prayer Answered

My name is Mary. I am a friend of Donald and Evelyn Daniel. I met this wonderful couple during Easter dinner at a mutual friend's home in 1997. This is significant in that my only son, Mark, was killed on June 8, 1996. Mark had left behind the joy of my life, my two-year-old grandson Micael.

At our first meeting, I remember Donald as a frail old man who had suffered a stroke and had difficulty with speech and getting around. Micael was a sad little boy who had lost his daddy and did not understand why. My husband and I explained to Donald and Evelyn that Micael did not talk much and certainly would not acknowledge any attention given on their part.

We finished dinner and helped Donald to the sofa to watch TV while we chatted over coffee at the table. No matter where I am or what I'm doing, I am aware of Micael. My eyes are drawn to him constantly. I noticed Micael place his hand on Donald's knee and then gently lean against his leg. As Donald watched this little one, the sweetest smile spread across Donald's face and a twinkle appeared in his eye. They started to chat about this and that, and before I knew it, Micael had brought out every toy he owned for Donald's inspection and approval.

I thought, WOW, none of our overwhelming love for Micael had reached him, but Donald's warmth, intelligence, and understanding had. Even in his weakened state, this wonderful soul knew instinctively what to say and do for this precious child. It was then and there that I fell in love with the Daniels.

We saw each other only two more times before I received a call from a grief-stricken Evelyn. Her precious love had been diagnosed with Alzheimer's. She does not remember, but we had many late night telephone conversations. By this time, I had lost my beloved husband of twenty-five years. He followed our son to the grave. He could not bear to live without him.

And then, Donald Daniel passed away. Evelyn called to invite me to his memorial service. It was a beautiful service that celebrated Donald's life. As I sat listening to "Evelyn's kids" talk about "Papa," I wished that I could have known him better.

After the service, I kept in touch with Evelyn, stopping by on my way home from work. I watched with great alarm as enormous grief drained her life away.

I prayed for guidance and wisdom to find a way to help Evelyn. All I could do was to sit and listen.

Not long after, Evelyn asked if she could come and live with me.

I knew then that my prayers had been answered.

MARY S. BARRASS

Is it C.R.S. or Alzheimer's?

I remember when it began. My sister and I were leaving a restaurant seven miles from my home. She was driving, and as we laughed about childhood experiences, I noticed she had difficulty staying in her lane on the freeway. She also missed the exit to my house. We chalked passing the exit to talking too much and not paying attention. We both laughed about it.

"Everyone has had this experience at least once in her life. Besides, we're getting on in age and _Can't Remember Stuff_," I told her. I am sixty-eight and she is seven years older.

One night, a few weeks later, my brother-in-law called to ask if my sister had come to visit me. I live in Acton, California and she lives in Central Los Angeles.

"Of course not. She is not with me," I said.

Then he confessed that she'd driven to the market less than a mile away, and after five hours, had not returned home.

During our conversation, I learned that there had been other times she'd been missing for hours, and when she had told him she could not find her way home.

I was still not aware that anything was wrong. I'd often been upset with my husband and taken long drives to avoid an argument. I figured my sister wanted to do the same, since she had marital problems.

They were a typical "keep up with the Joneses" family and eventually purchased a three-bedroom townhouse in suburban

Atlanta, Georgia, where they spent time during the spring and fall. During one of these visits, my niece called me late at night from Georgia, crying that her daughter and my sister had been missing for several hours after driving to the corner restaurant to pick up their take-out dinners.

An easily excitable woman in her forties, I calmed my niece enough to learn that just she, her young daughter with cerebral palsy, and my sister had taken a vacation without her father, my sister's husband.

I asked my niece for a description of the rental car and what her daughter and my sister were wearing. I then told her to wait by the phone. I called the Atlanta missing persons division and told them that my sister was missing and that she had Alzheimer's disease. This way, they would not wait for the standard twenty-four hours before searching for two adults.

Within two hours, the Atlanta police called to say that the Alabama law enforcement had apprehended a disoriented driver who fit the description—more than eighty miles away.

Months later, during a family reunion in Las Vegas, Nevada, my husband and I, and two of our four adult children, rented double suites in Circus Circus Hotel's tower to use as hospitality rooms for arriving relatives. My sister, who rode with us, rented a room in the lower bungalow next to the room in which my brother would be staying. He was due to arrive from Pittsburgh, Pennsylvania within the hour. I went with her to her room and then promptly went up to the suites to set them up.

My brother's plane had a mechanical problem and had to return to Pittsburgh for repairs. Unknown to us at the time, he would arrive more than eight hours late. After he checked into his room he realized he could not find our sister.

After calling hotel security, which checked her room, we learned that she had not unpacked and had not slept in her bed. After we searched everywhere with no success we called the local police for help. Within an hour they found my sister at the MGM hotel, five miles away. She had walked there to find me and to assist with the reunion, except this was the reunion we had four years earlier for the other side of our family.

It was then that Brenda Avadian's book, *"Where's my shoes?" My Father's Walk Through Alzheimer's,* really hit home. My sister had shut out the present and was living in the past. It sure seemed like my sister had Alzheimer's, especially the way Brenda's book described it.

I told my brother-in-law what I suspected. His reply was unsettling. "You've got a problem on your hands," he said.

"What do you mean, I've got a problem?" I demanded.

"She never cared nothing about me, so why should I care about her now?" he snapped.

I blew a fuse and threatened him with every law I could think of. I demanded copies of her medical coverage so that I could have her medical condition diagnosed.

Despite the fact that my sister has a husband and two adult children, I decided to help her and drove the 120-miles round trip each time she had an appointment. She is my only sister, and I love her. Perhaps most important is how she reached out to me when I was torn apart after graduating from high school in 1950 in our hometown of Pittsburgh.

❧   ❧   ❧

My parents were just getting by and raising eight children. The six who preceded me never finished high school. I worked hard to maintain a 4.0 grade point average to make my parents proud. I was overjoyed when I received an academic scholarship for four years at Duquesne University in Pittsburgh. But when I arrived to register, I saw the look of surprise on the registrar's face. I was told that my intellectual background was not high enough to attend their university.

My sister rescued me. She brought me to Los Angeles to live with her. She registered me at California State University-Los Angeles where the only costs were registration fees and books.

❧   ❧   ❧

After several weeks, I received the results of my sister's medical exams. She has glaucoma and diabetes. She had a stroke and her dementia is advanced to the point that she is no longer able to drive and can no longer be alone.

Her husband is trying his best to help her now, but she has become quite a handful with her strange behaviors.

One of these is pilfering. While visiting us, she took my husband's hearing aids. It wasn't until weeks later that my brother-in-law found them in *his* car. Often when we go shopping, my sister becomes combative or tries to leave the store without paying. She also curses like a drunken sailor. I thought she'd enjoy a shopping trip to Wal-Mart, until she cursed me as loudly as she could scream. Embarrassed, I left her alone until I finished my shopping. I found her at the security station where they'd ushered her. She was trying to leave with a full shopping cart of items. I explained her condition and lied about her wandering off and getting lost.

Whenever I visit her she asks how our mother is doing. Mom died almost a year and a half ago.

She puts on several layers of clothing and sometimes wears her left shoe on her right foot and her right shoe on her left foot.

When I take her to a buffet-style restaurant, she picks at the food with her fingers and eats it while standing there.

My sister has steadily advanced well-beyond C.R.S., but it fills my heart with joy to finally be able to give back to her the loving care that she gave to me so many years ago.

EULA YOUNGBLOOD

David's Pink Purse

It was a Saturday afternoon and members of our Toastmasters Club were gathered at our home. The occasion was our annual picnic. This year's theme: "High Desert Toastmasters Go to Tahiti!"

David and I wanted to travel to Tahiti for a relaxing vacation, but we never made it. So we brought Tahiti to the High Desert of Southern California. This would take some doing—we live at the southwestern edge of the Mojave Desert.

We decorated our home and the outdoors with brightly colored tropical birds, dancing girls in grass skirts, plastic tropical fish, framed tropical photos, tropical clothing, shell necklaces, and of course, tiki torches. We brought Tahiti to the California desert and we were ready for FUN.

❦   ❦   ❦

Our Toastmasters group was founded over thirty years ago by a lovely couple, Paris and Lucille, who were, until recently, very active with the club. Approaching their early eighties and facing health problems, they were unable to be as active. During the last few years, the club grew, representing countries from around the world. Our members' ages range from the thirties to mid-eighties. The one thing that has never changed is how we welcome guests and members. Visitors tell us that they feel very welcome in our club. We credit Lucille and Paris with providing the anchor for the club for so many years.

❧   ❧   ❧

Despite their declining health, Lucille and Paris surprised us by accepting our invitation to *Tahiti*. (Paris has difficulty breathing due to emphysema. Lucille has vascular dementia—a cruel memory-robbing disease for a very sweet woman.)

But they made the trek to our home (about an hour's drive). Lucille arrived, wearing a dressy white blouse and black slacks. In the spirit of the tropical occasion, she carried a bright fluorescent pink purse.

As Lucille and Paris made themselves comfortable on the double recliner in our family room, I noticed Lucille holding onto her purse. Frequently she looked inside, pulling out one thing then another. She'd examine it and then return the item to her purse. She held her purse close and when she got up to get food it hung awkwardly from her arm. When she went to the bathroom she took it with her. Feeling that it was awkward for her, I offered to place it on our bed where it would be safe and she could easily retrieve it if she needed it. She said, "Okay" and then held onto it tightly. Thinking she misunderstood my offer, I repeated it. This time she said, "No thank you" and extended her arm to hand it to me. I smiled, took her purse, and placed it on the bed.

As more guests arrived, David and I, already wearing our flower leis, handed each guest a colorful lei.

Once most of our guests had arrived we enjoyed an abundance of food. Each family brought a dish that represented their culture. We enjoyed international cuisine and great *conversation*. After all, *we are Toastmasters!*

As some people got up for second and third helpings, I noticed Lucille's purse on her lap. I watched as she took out an item, looked at it, and then returned it to her purse. She did this several times and then closed her purse and placed it by her side.

After people had eaten their fill, some of the club officers started conducting business. *Can't anyone stop talking about work at a party?*

A while later, Paris and Lucille said it would be best if they got ready to leave since it was getting dark outside and they had a long drive home. David and I helped them gather their things.

❦ ❦ ❦

Frequently, following our Toastmaster meetings, Lucille would leave something behind. Once she left her reading glasses. I sent them to her by priority mail. A couple of times, she left her purse. While a few of us stayed and chatted after the meetings, she and Paris returned for her purse.

❦ ❦ ❦

Knowing they might leave something behind, I asked David to make sure they had everything before they left.

We scurried about, going back and forth—in the kitchen, on the love seat in the living room where people had placed their things, and in the bedroom. We wanted to be sure Paris and Lucille had taken everything they brought with them. Once we were assured nothing was left, we helped carry their things to their car. We bid them farewell and returned to the party. It was then I saw it … Lucille's pink purse!

David said he'd try to catch them on foot. He grabbed the purse and dashed hastily out the front door before I thought to say anything. I returned to the business meeting, which by now was in full swing. And then my mind began to wander … a man running down the street at night wearing a red T-shirt, black shorts, a flower lei, clutching onto a bright pink purse. I smiled at this image (like I am doing right now) and then couldn't contain myself. Apologizing for interrupting the meeting, I described my vision. The Toastmasters laughed uproariously.

Soon after David returned, gasping. He was still wearing the flower lei and clutching the pink purse. He had not been successful in catching up with Lucille and Paris, so he decided to go after them in *my* car—thinking that Paris would recognize my car if it pulled along side him. Now, one minor detail bears mentioning. My car was serviced at the dealer and we picked it up the afternoon before. Since then, I had not driven it.

Once David pulled out of the garage he realized that the headlights did not work—we learned later the mechanic forgot to re-install the fuse. Meanwhile, as I walked past the counter where David kept his wallet, I noticed his wallet was still there. So, again, while the Toastmasters conducted their business meeting in *Tahiti* I imagined my husband driving *my* car on the freeway wearing a flower lei, with no identification, except for that *pink purse* by his side on the passenger seat. I further imagined him being stopped, asked for identification, and then being detained in the local jail for suspicion of theft—of my car and Lucille's purse.

I could not stop laughing and once more interrupted the Toastmasters. I shared this second vision. This time they stopped the meeting and joined in the laughter. "Sure, we'll come with you to post bail," they said. One added, "When we see David behind bars we'll enthusiastically exclaim, 'Hi, Lucille! What happened? And where's your pink purse?' "

While we laughed at his expense, David returned, carrying Lucille's pink purse. We teased him and, in his good-natured spirit, he joined our laughter. That's when we learned the headlights didn't work.

When we considered the penalties—stolen car, stolen purse, and the lights not working … well, this just made us laugh all the more!

I called and left a message on Lucille's and Paris' answering machine. The following day Paris called and suggested we get together for lunch. We did and laughed again as we recounted David's adventures of the night before.

Now, Lucille has her pink purse.

BRENDA AVADIAN, MA
The Caregiver's Voice

SECTION V

Celebrations

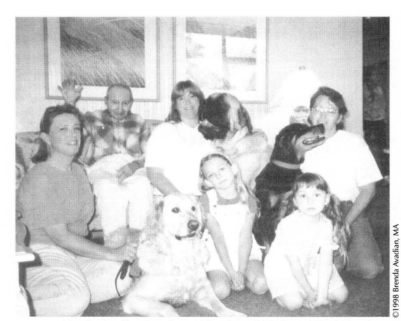

Martin Avadian (waving) with a few of his furry friends
and their handlers.

Celebrations are as important to people with Alzheimer's and their families as they are to anyone else. They can be festive occasions with all the decorations or they can be simple moments in time.

In December 1999, I sent an e-mail reply to Marilyn, a fellow author who inquired about my father. I wrote, "Each moment that I share with my father is a celebration of life, which gets increasingly difficult as he enters more deeply into his own world, moving away from the world as we have come to know it."

Months earlier, on a warm and gentle breezy July afternoon, the aides helped the residents outside to enjoy the nice weather. When David and I arrived, they were reading movie trivia questions. Many of the old-timers answered them correctly. My father, who had difficulty hearing, sat near two aides. Even though he didn't answer any of the questions, he seemed to enjoy everyone else's responses and laughter.

David and I arrived with a few miniature 3 Musketeers® candy bars. My father loved anything that was "easy on the teeth" and sweet. We gave one to him and he savored it. He opened his mouth for more. When he finished the second candy bar, one of the aides asked him how he liked the candy. I think he came up with a new slogan for 3 Musketeers®. He said, "Sure beats cancer holes!" Where this response came from was beyond any of us. We all laughed heartily, and my father, seeing us enjoying ourselves, joined in.

I couldn't resist. When I got home, I sent an e-mail to June Kolf, a friend and an author, whose husband was battling bladder cancer. I suggested she get him to try this new cancer cure that my father had discovered. She sent me a short e-mail and closed it with, "Gotta go and give my husband a 3 Musketeers® candy bar."

Celebrations include the special occasions we will remember for a long time. Sometimes they are brief, like the lucid moment Debbie Center's mother had in "Ice Cream Never Tasted so Good." Other times, they involve family members' reactions to unfulfilled expectations, as in Kay Runner's "Slept Right Through Thanksgiving."

Celebrations may involve carefully orchestrated reunions that result in a long-term effect upon a family that has grown apart geographically, as in "Four Special Days" by Laurie Frasier.

Finally, Cindy Lester's account in "The Wedding" proves that you can have a memorable occasion among friends—even if your husband marries another woman on your anniversary.

Ice Cream Never Tasted So Good!

It had been nearly four years since the summer of 1996 when we realized something awful was happening to Mom. She began doing strange things, like pouring orange juice on her cereal and getting lost in familiar places. These symptoms came on so suddenly that doctors believed Mom had been suffering from small TIA strokes. Recently, however, they began to suspect she may have Alzheimer's disease.

I feel as though Mom is like a beautiful butterfly, trapped in the cocoon of a body that Alzheimer's has aggressively transformed into nothing more than a shell of the person we love so much. Thankfully there are still moments when Alzheimer's disease seems to disappear, just long enough for us to catch a glimpse of Mom's beautiful inner spirit, which still lives inside of her. I think that we are allowed these glimpses so that we never forget that our loved one is still in there somewhere, begging for our help. We must never lose sight of the fact that they're still with us, if only for brief but treasured appearances.

We had such an appearance from Mom in April 2000. Her oldest sister had come from Pennsylvania to visit us in Colorado. One evening, about twelve members of our extended family were gathered in Mom's home, where she had lived for thirty-one years, twenty-five as a widow.

Her two oldest grandchildren had been living with her for over a year. They were a tremendous blessing for Mom, helping her with meals, cleaning, companionship, etc. We had also hired a neighbor, a Certified Nurse's Aide, to come twice a day to help Mom. This once fiercely independent woman was now completely dependent on those around her for assistance with all activities of daily living, as the pros call it.

This evening, however, was one to be remembered. As we were gathered in the living room, Mom was sitting rather listlessly on the couch. We couldn't help but wonder if she was aware that those who loved her so dearly surrounded her.

Suddenly Mom perked up and asked if anyone would like some ice cream. My children were thrilled by the offer, and, as I was about to go into the kitchen to get the dishes of ice cream, Mom beat me to the punch!

She quickly went into the kitchen with the children. The rest of us just sat there, staring at one another in awe, wondering what was happening. As Mom bustled about in the kitchen, we later learned that she was looking for the ice cream in the cupboard. That's dementia for you! My son quickly led her to the freezer and Mom pulled out the ice cream. She then took out four bowls and spoons, scooped four bowls of ice cream, and served ice cream to my children, herself, and me!

She then asked if anyone else would like some. All this from a woman who hadn't served anything to anyone in years! I shed tears of joy and offered many prayers of thanks as I ate the best ice cream I'd ever tasted in my life!

You just never know when your loved one will make a guest appearance, shoving their way out of the cocoon and into your heart once again.

DEBBIE CENTER
Piano Teacher

Slept Through Thanksgiving

In 1995 my husband, George, and I had been retired for eight years. Although George ran a small electrical business during retirement, we enjoyed our home, our grandchildren, and traveling in our RV. Just before Christmas, we received a call from my ninety-year-old mother in Florida. She said she didn't want to live alone any longer. (My father had passed away in 1990.) We went to Florida to discuss her options.

We decided to share her care with family. My brother would spend time with her in Florida, and then our mother would live with relatives in New York and California. Eventually Mom could no longer continue this routine, so George and I chose to have her live with us in California.

At first Mother joined us at our church and community activities. And she also helped campaign for our son, who was running for state legislator. Later though, she started getting confused and stopped enjoying these activities. I didn't know what to do for her. I needed information and support, so I called the Alzheimer's Association. They referred me to the Visiting Nurse Adult Day Care Center support group in Lancaster, California.

At the support group, when I explained my situation, they suggested I have my mother evaluated at the Center for Aging Research and Evaluation at the Granada Hills Community Hospital. I did, and that was when we learned she was suffering from Alzheimer's. Our lives would not be the same.

We received outstanding comfort and support from the support group. George and I also attended an Alzheimer's conference in Pasadena, which helped us better understand the disease. Still, we were unprepared for many situations.

One, in particular, is quite memorable to this day.

The year was 1997. Thanksgiving was fast approaching. Mom was having trouble sleeping at night, so she slept a lot during the day. I wanted her to enjoy Thanksgiving with our family of four children, nine grandchildren, and a nephew who was flying in to see his grandma, so I asked our pharmacist if he could recommend something to help her sleep through the night. This way she would be awake to enjoy Thanksgiving. He suggested Benadryl® as a mild sleeping aid.

The night before Thanksgiving we helped get Mom settled. We were looking forward to a good night's sleep ourselves when she popped up, looking like she was ready to party. The medicine had a reverse reaction on her. Needless to say, we were up all night. When the sun rose Mom finally fell asleep. She looked so peaceful. We proceeded to get ready for our big outing.

After a while we realized the medicine had finally kicked in. For the next two hours we tried to wake her. We had her drink black coffee. We put her in her wheelchair and walked her up and down the sidewalk in front of our home. (We hoped the neighbors would not come out and ask what we had done to this poor sweet lady who was sleeping through all of this!) It was obvious Mom was not going to wake up. We had no option but to dress her, put her in the car, and head to our son's home for a wonderful Thanksgiving that I had wanted my mom to enjoy.

It was a surprise to our family when George and I carried Grandma in and laid her on the couch. This day was not going as I had planned. Everyone was busy getting ready for the turkey to come out of the oven. We tried to get Mom in a safe and what we thought would be a comfortable position. Her great-grandchildren covered her with a favorite blanket and propped a large stuffed animal on her lap. This would be her position for the rest of the day.

There was Mom (Grandma, Great Grandma) sleeping in the chair as we enjoyed dinner, dessert, table talk, and games.

As the sun was setting, Mom began to wake up. She hadn't eaten all day, so we propped her up at the table and encouraged her to eat, like a parent would a baby. After much coaxing, she opened her mouth and began to eat. But she still had her eyes closed! We bragged about her eating and how good the food was. She smiled, enjoying every bite … with her eyes closed.

It was wonderful how the family joined in and enjoyed having her there, just the way she was.

When the time came for us to leave, as we were walking out the door, someone asked, "Wasn't the turkey great, Grandma?"

She replied, "I didn't have any turkey."

This was the beginning of many funny, and also difficult, adventures with my mother on her walk with Alzheimer's.

KAY RUNNER

Four Special Days

My mother has Alzheimer's. It is a tragedy and a nightmare that has changed my life. Alzheimer's has impacted every family member and friend I have. It is woven into my thoughts and conversations. It affects my daily schedule and my plans for the future. Although my mother is the one who has Alzheimer's, both of us are victims of this ugly disease.

Despite its ugliness, Alzheimer's has given me a gift, which has brought me incredible joy and comfort. I feel both happy and lucky due to Alzheimer's. It was two summers ago, in early June, that this joyous gift became apparent to me.

As Alzheimer's advanced and my mother became less able to take care of herself, I moved her from Dallas, Texas (her home of forty years) to Grand Junction, Colorado—800 miles away from her family and friends. It was a necessary move because it made it possible for me to give her the care she needed. It was a good thing; yet, I felt terribly guilty for doing this to her. So, I wanted to do something that would make her very happy. I decided to have a June family reunion in her honor.

My mother has two brothers and one sister, with accompanying sisters and brothers-in-law; a passel of nieces and nephews, and their kids. There were a total of twenty-eight. I made phone calls and sent letters. Would they be willing to come to Colorado for a big surprise family reunion in honor of Mom, knowing that time with her was now a precious commodity? They all said, "Yes."

They rearranged their lives and work schedules to attend. For most, it was an 800-mile journey. Some would drive; others would fly.

One cousin flew in from Florida with her five-year-old daughter, Leila, who since birth had Dejerrine-Sotas, a very rare form of muscular dystrophy. This meant she had to bring all of Leila's equipment—power wheelchair, oxygen, medications, etc. This would be a miracle in itself.

I kicked into major planning mode. I made arrangements. This reunion was to be a four-day extravaganza like no other.

We have always been a close family, but as time passed and everyone grew older and spread out to various parts of the country, we spent less time together. Phone calls were rare. The reunion gave everyone a new sense of purpose and a reason to call or e-mail. We were doing this for Mom. We were doing this because we were family.

It was incredibly fun and exciting to plan this reunion. I made "to do" lists, an itinerary, and even commemorative T-shirts. I booked hotel rooms, restaurants, caterers, a van, a rafting excursion, and a musician. I assigned duties and planned special awards. I even set up a special "Memory Presentation," which required everyone's participation. There was no detail left unplanned. This was to be a once-in-a-lifetime event. It was all I could do to keep it a surprise for my mom!

The big weekend finally arrived and so did family. The next four days were remarkable.

The big event of the first night included the Memory Presentations. Each person came prepared with a story, a song, or a poem—something special to be shared in front of and remembered by all—a special memory of Mom, Dad, or grandparents who were no longer with us. Tears flowed freely during the Memory Presentations. The poignancy was overwhelming. We watched and listened to each other, in awe of the moment and of the memories.

The time sped by as we ate, drank, laughed, and cried.

We talked about Mom's health deteriorating when she wasn't within hearing range.

We watched Leila drive up and down the street in her wheelchair, with the other kids on roller blades, hanging on like a train.

We crammed into vehicles and drove over to the Colorado National Monument. We posed for each other's cameras, like tourists. We delighted in the beauty of the scenery, not to mention we all looked spiffy together in our matching commemorative T-shirts.

We played dominos and cards—a family tradition—at a park down by the river, and cheered Aunt Kaye when she beat her brothers in the domino tournament.

We laughed when my two cousins and two sisters, got in a catfight and called each other the "b" word.

We ate catfish in memory of Pappy, my grandfather. We had Cousins-Night-Out-on-the-Town-While-the-Old-Fogeys-Stay-Home-and-Baby-sit-the-Grandkids Night.

We went river rafting—a new experience for most.

We were entertained by and sang along with my friend Lloyd, a fabulous singer and guitarist, who performed a special concert for us. Uncle Kirk sang, "Hey Good Looking." We had never heard him sing before. Uncle Robert and Mom, fondly known as "Dude and Sarah" sang a duet, one we all knew well, because we had heard them sing it for years. Uncle Robert said it was the last time it was to be sung. Uncle Butch and Uncle Robert sang. Jim, Julie, and my son, Caleb sang. Spencer, Dustin, Leila, and Cyndi sang.

It was both amazing and delightful.

Sadly, the weekend came to an end. We finished with a goodbye brunch and awards for all.

Those four days changed my life. They taught me that there is nothing stronger and more precious and uplifting than the love and support of family. The ugliness of Alzheimer's had brought all of us together for a four-day feast of bonding and reconfirmation of love. We all felt it. We all thrived on it.

Shortly after the Colorado reunion, five-year-old Leila, passed away. We cherish the memory of the Colorado reunion all the more, knowing we were truly blessed with her presence on those four very special days.

❧   ❧   ❧

The reunion was two years ago, but the phone calls and e-mails continue. This is my gift and my greatest joy. My family calls to find out how Mom is doing and to tell me how much they love me. They tell me how proud they are of my strength and how much they miss me. They call to remind me that we are now committed to having a reunion each year.

Uncle Butch held it in Austin this past summer. Aunt Kaye will have it in Lubbock next summer. Meanwhile, we have reunited for other events and mini get-togethers.

As is often the case in life, my family had drifted apart. Alzheimer's brought us together again, with joy … with strength … with love.

LAURIE FRASIER

The Wedding

Last June we held a mock wedding at Daybreak, a group activity and respite program for persons suffering from memory disorders. This wedding brought back many cherished memories. It was a joyous event, not only for our participants, but for our families, staff, and friends as well.

We prepared for this magic day by asking our participants' family members' permission to have their loved ones in the wedding. Our goal was to include all participants in the wedding, in whatever way best suited them. This was critical in determining who would be our bride and groom. Since both of the chosen participants had been married before, we didn't want to cause any miscomprehension such as, "What do you mean? I'm getting married again?"

After our bride and groom were selected, we let the bride decide on the color scheme for the mock wedding. She also wanted to select her next husband!!!!! We then chose a best man and maid of honor.

The rest of the participants stood up for the bride and groom as our bridesmaids and groomsmen. At the last minute we even asked the bus driver to give our bride away!! My minister's daughter made a wedding cake, which doubled as her 4-H project. She also agreed to be our flower girl. Families were asked to bring the participants' memoirs and pictures of their own weddings, which we displayed on the table near the altar.

Our staff pitched in where needed, from flower arranging (from our personal garden) to a mock minister, and taking our bride-to-be out the day before to treat her to a facial and a hair and nail makeover. The beauty shop even donated beautiful diamond earrings to the cause.

With our personal funny vows at hand, the wedding began and ended with a lot of laughter. We shared precious memories, and the pretend bride and groom stole the show.

It was a joyous occasion that all will remember forever.

❦   ❦   ❦

As we reminisced, a past participant's wife, Sandy Petri, shared the following: "My husband was diagnosed with Alzheimer's at the age of fifty-two. That was eleven years ago, and I find the little funny stories help me get through. A year ago, as we were getting into bed, my husband said that he thought we should get married. At first I was upset that he didn't remember we were married, but then I thought it was great that after thirty-seven years, he still wanted to marry me. When I told my sisters, they teased me, 'You are living in sin.' The following June, the Daybreak program—without which I could not have kept my husband at home as long as I did—said they were having a mock wedding. One of the participants wanted to marry my husband (the strangest thing is that her youngest son dated our daughter in high school). The director of Daybreak invited me to attend. When I asked the date, she said, 'June sixteenth.' I exclaimed, 'Oh no, that is our anniversary!' Not only did he not remember we were married, but now he was going to be married to another woman on our anniversary! I suggested they have him as best man to avoid more confusion. The mock wedding was fun and I enjoyed being there."

❦   ❦   ❦

The groom's daughter, Pat Hahn, said, "It is difficult to communicate with my father because he repeats himself many times. However, the one thing he repeats that I know is sincere is, 'I love you and don't you ever forget that!' "

CINDY LESTER
Program Coordinator, DAYBREAK

SECTION VI

The Birds and the Bees

What were *you* expecting?

This is a *family* book!

I toyed with the idea of titling this section, "<u>A</u> to <u>X</u>: The beginning of <u>A</u>lzheimer's does not mean the end of se<u>x</u>." It is comforting to know that as people age they still have the desire to, and DO, light the candles of passion, love, and romance.

Despite the forgetfulness due to Alzheimer's, couples that overcome the initial shock of not being recognized by their partners, grow to accept the disease for what it is. Some toy with the freshness this uncertainty brings, as Helen did in "You'd better go now, my wife will be home soon."

The key to coping is knowing what to expect. These family members learned as much as they could about this disease and attended support group meetings. They were able to accept the inevitable progress of Alzheimer's as Evelyn Daniel and Marion Riley share in their stories, "Lovers for Fifty-Six Years" and "A Bedtime Story."

Children, who lovingly care for their parents with Alzheimer's, sometimes have to fight back their surprise and show understanding when Mom or Dad asks a direct question. Gil Lozano is placed in a delicate position with his mother in "Do I have Erectile Dysfunction?" Jeanne Parsons, who usually has little difficulty expressing herself, is left speechless after her mother asks, "I forget dear, what's an orgasm?" And when a family friend decides to get married, Dr. Marlene Caroselli will admit eyebrows raised with "The Naked Bride."

"Do I have Erectile Dysfunction?"

Remember the Pfizer television commercial that aired a while back? It first showed a disease or illness, followed by the Pfizer product that could help alleviate the problem. First the disease would pan across the screen (Alzheimer's), then the Pfizer product would follow (Aricept®). Five or more products panned across the screen in the same manner, including erectile dysfuntion and Viagra®.

One Saturday evening, Gil Lozano, a first-generation Hispanic American and retired aerospace engineer, sat with his ninety-year-old mother, who has Alzheimer's, in her East L.A. home of forty-plus years. They were watching television when this Pfizer commercial appeared.

Gil was his mom's primary caregiver for weeks at a time, and it was his nature to make it a fun experience for the two of them. When he saw "Alzheimer's" pan across the screen he turned to his mom and said, "Look, Mom, that's the disease you have."

He watched her as she intently focused on the screen and began reading the words aloud, "Penile Erectile Dys..." Shocked, he quickly turned to the television to see "Viagra®" pan across the screen.

He started laughing. He didn't realize she could read so fast and actually pronounce the words.

He couldn't stop laughing. The thought of his ninety-year-old mother reading such words was too funny.

Then she turned to him and innocently asked, "Son, is *that* the disease I have?"

Gil couldn't contain himself. He laughed so hard he slipped off the couch onto the floor.

"She surprises me every time. I never know what to expect from her."

BASED ON A STORY BY GIL LOZANO
Retired Engineer

"You'd better go now, my wife will be home soon."

Helen was a dear friend to many caregivers who looked forward to her sense of humor and unique view of the world. Each time she came to the caregiver meetings or to our monthly luncheons she would ask a profound question. "If light travels at the speed of light, at what speed does dark travel?" The one that really had us talking was, "Did Adam and Eve have belly buttons?"

We knew Helen by three things—the hats she wore, her sense of humor, and her deep and abiding philosophies about the world. As often is the case, when Helen and I called each other, our "brief" conversations would extend for an hour or more. She was a great conversationalist and one who probed issues deeply.

And so it was that her second husband, Jim, became my father's roommate upon his admission to the skilled nursing facility. Jim was about six feet tall and weighed about 200 pounds. He quietly wandered the halls in stocking feet, minding his own business. He was a career pilot and, knowing a few while I worked in aerospace, I wondered what happens to these active, confident, and frequently cocky pilots who are struck down by this debilitating disease?

I would regularly greet him, "Hi Jim," to which he'd have a slight facial reaction. Then I'd say something about the planes he flew. Helen had taped pictures of them to the wall above the headboard of his bed. Jim would stop, look at me, try to recognize me, and then not knowing who I was, look down and shuffle along; going about his business.

As Alzheimer's took its toll on Jim's brain, he struggled to keep his balance. During one of his repeated falls, he broke his hip. Upon his return from the hospital, he was unable to walk and eventually caught an infection. He was moved to the non-ambulatory station, where wheelchair and bedridden residents reside.

Helen visited her husband regularly. As his health declined he became bedridden. Still, she tried to be playful with him— difficult given the circumstances of his physical misery and that he rarely said anything. She even brought in wine coolers for Jim to enjoy because they helped him relax. Helen was a true patient advocate; she wanted what was best for her husband. If the rules didn't make sense, like "No Alcohol," she questioned them until she was satisfied with the answer, or found a way around them, as was the case with the wine coolers.

❧   ❧   ❧

During one afternoon visit, she was in a playful mood and Jim seemed to be responsive. He took her hand and she placed her other hand on his shoulder. She bent over to give him a kiss and wanted to hold him. It was a little awkward to try and hold him as he lay in the bed. So she lay by his side and rested her arm on his chest. She spoke softly in his ear.

Jim relaxed for a while, then as if he had been deliberately shocked, he abruptly looked up. He tried to sit up and pulled his head away from this woman by his side. This man, who had not communicated in months, clearly said, "You'd better go now, my wife will be home soon. And I don't think she will appreciate seeing you here."

Helen pulled away from him enough to look at him in surprise. In her characteristic style she burst out laughing. Then she got off of the bed and now laughing in disbelief, packed her things to leave.

Feeling a sense of relief, Jim relaxed.

As Helen walked out the door, she added, "Okay, we don't want your wife to find out. I'll see you later."

"Hm-hm," came the reply.

BRENDA AVADIAN, MA
The Caregiver's Voice

(Author's Note: It was my honor and privilege to be Helen's friend. I dedicate this story to her memory. A strong and independent woman, sadly she passed away suddenly of an aneurysm and her husband followed her a few weeks later.)

Lovers for Fifty-Six Years

Once I grew more accustomed to Don's strange behavior, I was able to laugh *with* him. He had recently been diagnosed with Alzheimer's and was now living in a secured skilled nursing center specializing in dementia care.

One day, I walked into his room. He was not expecting me. When I saw the old familiar gleam in his eye, my heart lurched with joy.

He hugged me and kissed me again and again. Then, holding me close, he said, "I want to make love to you."

"Why not?" I thought. "We'd been lovers for fifty-six years! But where?"

His bed was one of three in the room and I told him we would not have much privacy.

Don then suggested I sign him out for a visit "home."

"Plenty good," I said, "sounds like a plan to me!"

So I drove us back to our apartment and we made love. Then I drove Don back to the care center.

On the way, he began to laugh and said, "I would have never believed my lady would drive forty miles for a piece of ass!"

So it seemed he did have some memory left.

EVELYN DANIEL

A Bedtime Story

My husband, Don, was diagnosed with Alzheimer's disease in 1992. He was sixty-seven years old and we had been married for forty-six years. We had many happy years together, we traveled a lot and, most of all, we enjoyed our grandchildren.

Don is an easygoing person with a quiet demeanor. When he said or did anything out of the ordinary, I had a hard time with it at first, but I knew I had to accept his condition. As the disease progressed he would do really odd and funny things.

He had been getting up at night and wouldn't come back to bed. One predawn morning at about 3:00, he decided to get up.

I was so tired of getting up with him each time, I stayed in bed and begged him, "Don, please come back to bed."

He was reluctant, yet as he crawled back into bed, he replied, "I don't think my wife would appreciate me going to bed with you!"

MARION RILEY

"I forget dear, what's an orgasm?"

My mother was a kind, patient, and caring person, with a wonderful sense of humor.

Alzheimer's is not fun for the patient or the caregiver. But in my experience, having a sense of humor made a difficult situation less difficult. The following are some of my recollections of caring for my mother.

※　　※　　※

The Grand Seduction

I started caring for my mother when my stepfather was hospitalized with kidney failure and then passed away. My mother was in the early stages of Alzheimer's. However, for several months she seemed confused about what had happened to my stepdad. She frequently mistook my husband for her late husband. One morning as my husband was reading the paper; she walked up to him and embraced his face with her very large breasts. My husband panicked and ran next door to our daughter's, and asked her what to do about his mother-in-law trying to seduce him. Our daughter calmed him down, but it took awhile.

※　　※　　※

Too Many Old People

Shortly thereafter we decided that my mother could use more socialization and stimulation in her life. She was seventy-nine.

We took her to the local adult day care center, where Mom met with some of the participants who were in their sixties and seventies, the staff, and caregivers. We observed several of their activities. Later, while driving home, I asked Mom what she thought about participating in the program. She said, "Well dear, it is very nice, but I prefer not to spend so much time around old people."

    ✳   ✳   ✳

What's An Orgasm?
About two years later I was sitting with my mother watching a PBS program on human sexuality. (Mom was still able to focus on some television programs.) She turned to me after a few minutes of watching and asked, "I forget dear, what's an orgasm?"

As I struggled to answer my eighty-one-year-old mother's question, I thought, Never did I imagine that this is what I would be doing at age fifty-seven! It became very clear at this moment that our roles were now certainly reversed.

When one takes care of a parent with Alzheimer's the reversal of roles can be very traumatic, but maintaining a healthy sense of humor can help ease the transition.

    ✳   ✳   ✳

She Is Much Nicer Than You Are
As Mom declined, she would get irritated with me when I'd redirect her from doing something unsafe, like walking outside by herself or using the stove without help.

One day when she was especially annoyed with my redirection she walked down the hall to the bathroom, and stood in front of the mirror. From where I was sitting, I could see her talking to her reflection in the mirror. A few minutes later she returned to me and said, "The lady in the bathroom is MUCH nicer than you are!"

❦   ❦   ❦

101 Uses For Shampoo, Use Number 86

When Mom was eighty-six, about six months before she passed away and when Alzheimer's had progressed toward the last stages, I continued to encourage her to participate in our daily activities. One day I was standing in the kitchen stirring a pot of fudge. Mom was standing beside me. I handed her the wooden spoon covered with fudge so she could lick it. (Mom loved chocolate.) I turned to pour the fudge into the pan, and looked back at Mom, who was smiling as she lovingly and carefully spread the fudge evenly through her hair. I was momentarily exasperated, when I thought, The most important thing happening here is that Mom is having fun. After all isn't that what shampoo is for?

❦   ❦   ❦

Sit Down and Shut Up (I Have One Nerve Left)

Near the end of my mother's battle with Alzheimer's she demonstrated one of the mysteries of the disease. Though she was mostly mute during this stage and responded very little to life around her, she could still walk as long as I walked with her.

Mom took to pacing almost constantly during the day, which meant I spent a good portion of the day pacing as well. As evening approached, this behavior would intensify, until sometimes she was up and pacing every three minutes.

Her doctor had prescribed several types of medications to help relax her. But none of them seemed to help at this stage.

One night, after many weeks of this behavior, I was growing more and more exasperated and exhausted. All my efforts to calm her did not work. My frustration level nearly did me in, and I snapped at her, "Mom, I have only one nerve left and you are standing on it. Please sit down for at least five minutes or I'll go crazy."

She looked at me more clearly than she had in several months and in an angry tone asked, "Would you like to trade places with me?"

I was stunned. All I could say was, "No, Mom. I'm sorry."

"WELL THEN SIT DOWN AND SHUT UP!"

How she could have expressed herself so clearly at this late stage in her disease will always be a mystery to me. Despite the anger we shared at the time, this memory makes me smile.

Mom could still share a little piece of her sense of humor with me after all.

JEANNE PARSONS

The Naked Bride

Francine became a part of our family through marriage, but the love she engendered could not have been stronger had our blood run in her veins. We visited her often in the nursing home and were pleased to find her lucid and even optimistic on the days when Alzheimer's made her live in the past rather than in the present.

She was ninety-five when she died, and she told my mom about her marital intentions during the last year of her life.

On one especially memorable day, my mother, who has sewn wedding gowns all of her life, was engaged in a conversation with Francine—a conversation rooted in the past but surprisingly oriented to the future.

"You know," she whispered conspiratorially, "I'm going to get married again."

And indeed, there was a certain resident, a man with a mysterious bag, who had caught her eye.

"That's wonderful, Francine," my mother replied, bestowing early congratulations.

"Yes," Francine asserted her intentions. "But *this* time, you don't have to make my wedding gown."

"Why not, Francine?" my mother inquired.

"Because this time," she declared with a girlish giggle, "I'm going to get married naked!"

DR. MARLENE CAROSELLI
Center for Professional Development

SECTION VII

Discoveries in Nursing Homes

One November afternoon in 1999, when my father was still able to draw on his sense of humor, I pulled out a mirror and held it in front of his face.

"See that face?" I asked. As my father looked at his reflection, I joked, "That's a face only a mother could love."

While continuing to stare at his reflection he replied with the greatest of sincerity, "A mother couldn't be that discreet."

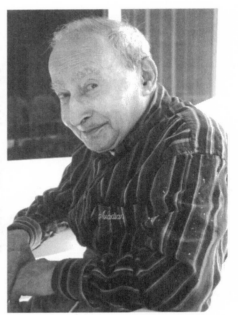

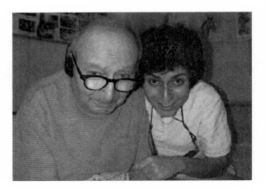

Martin Avadian hamming it up with his daughter Brenda during one of her visits to the nursing home.

Visiting a nursing home is one of those "growth" experiences. We learn to look beneath the surface and find the gifts. After a loved one is admitted, it takes a lot of strength for a caregiver, family member, or friend, to visit.

Initially, we feel guilty for placing them, and then we feel bad when we don't visit as often as we think we should. Fortunately, love, and sometimes a sense of duty, tug at us.

Some walk through the front door and enter a well-appointed home-away-from-home, as is the case with many assisted living communities and residential care facilities.

Others walk through the doors of a nursing home that offers a greater level of care. These facilities can be a harsh contrast to the assisted living communities because these residents need skilled nursing care. The care center where my father lived is such a place. A great number of their residents are in wheelchairs or recline in Geri-chairs, and visitors notice the occasional odor of cleaning solution.

I remember the early days in 1997 when my husband and I would cringe as we walked up the ramp to the outside door. We asked one another, "Do you think there will come a day when we get used to this?" Going through the locked double doors we would be thrust into another world of smells, sounds, and faces. "Why," we'd ask, "do these people live? How will our society deal with the increasing number of people who will fill these nursing homes in the future? Why do we choose to perpetuate lives of the 'living dead' as some call them?" Neither of us would want to live this way; nor do most people we ask.

Despite these perceived negatives, the fact is that over one million of our loved ones live in nursing homes and are given twenty-four hours of care—something we would not be able to provide ourselves.

So, we make a choice. We learn to accept this as another one of life's growing experiences. Many of us adapt our schedules and visit our loved ones regularly.

I visited my father as often as my schedule allowed—sometimes once a week, sometimes twice. I realized that once he was gone, I would no longer have this choice. Although he did not know me and didn't seem to react to my visits, I spent time with him knowing that if I were in his shoes, I would want my family or friends to remember and visit me, just like Marian writes in "A Hug, A Tender Touch." Besides, I was able to actively participate in his care. Most of all, I continued to learn the very essence of life with each visit. These are not the "living dead." These are people who have interests, loves, memories, and desires.

With the complexities and excessive materialism in life today, what a pleasure it is to bring someone joy by simply holding his or her hand, or rubbing a sore shoulder, or bringing in a little treat, like pudding or a chocolate candy bar. They are so thankful when we just spend time with them. Even if they don't show it, I know in my heart they feel better for it. They can teach us so much if we are willing to take the time to learn. These are the gifts found in nursing homes. And these are the reasons many of us visit.

Church groups, therapy dogs, family and friends, and especially children, walk through the doors to bring much pleasure to those inside.

What a joy it was to sing a song that was deeply etched in one man's mind in "Never to be Forgotten." What an exciting time it was for the daughter who presented her mother with a special gift in "The Victorian Tea Party." What a wonderful opportunity to learn life-long lessons in "Generation to Generation." And we cannot overlook the animals in our lives when one dog accomplishes something no caregiver had in years in "A Golden Retriever Makes a Difference."

Those who visit may bring gifts, but they leave with an even bigger gift in their hearts, knowing the tremendous joy their visit brought to those who cannot care for themselves.

Never to be Forgotten

For those who were there, it is a moment frozen in time, never to be forgotten.

It was my father's ninetieth birthday, and about thirty people had gathered at the Alzheimer's care center where he lives to celebrate with him. He seemed unusually bright and cheery as he was greeted, hugged, and loved by his wife, his brother, four of his eight children and numerous grandchildren and great-grandchildren. His brightest smile came when he saw his eldest surviving son, Dick, for the first time in three years. Although he couldn't articulate what he was feeling, you could just see the flash of recognition and feel the wave of emotion.

There were lots of photos, a couple of brief speeches, a little entertainment, and, of course, birthday cake and ice cream. Dad seemed to enjoy it all, especially the cake and ice cream.

Suddenly, it was time to go. No one was anxious to leave—least of all Dad—but mealtime at the care center was fast approaching, and we needed to clear the dining room. There was just time for one more rousing chorus of "Happy Birthday to You."

"No, wait," someone suggested. "Let's sing something that Dad can sing with us."

On the surface, that seemed ludicrous. Although Dad was quite alert through the event, coherent expression from him was limited to two- and three-word sentences: "I'm fine," "How are you?" and "Oh, no." He couldn't remember the names of those nearest and dearest to him; asking him to participate in a sing-along was an exercise in futility.

Wasn't it?

A different song was selected, one of Dad's favorites from years gone by: "Let Me Call You Sweetheart." Just the mention of the song was enough to evoke tender feelings from those of us who remember the many times it was sung at family gatherings and as a way of passing the time during long family trips. In my mind, I can still hear the melodic blending of Dad's bold and brassy bass with Mom's rich alto resonating in the old Impala as we musically made our way across the California desert to visit family members on the coast.

All eyes were focused on Dad as we began singing:

"Let me call you Sweetheart, I'm in love with you."

His lips began forming the words of lyrics indelibly etched somewhere in his mind.

"Let me hear you whisper that you love me, too."

His eyebrows arched. His eyes sparkled.

"Keep the love light burning in your eyes so blue."

I was kneeling close to him, and could hear him singing. It wasn't the strong, vibrant voice that had embarrassed me as it boomed out mercilessly in countless church meetings through the years. But it was unmistakably Dad's voice.

"Let me call you Sweetheart, I'm in love with you."

He smiled happily as we harmoniously reached the end of the song.

Tears moistened most eyes as we savored the magic of the moment. For a few measures, at least, Dad was Dad again, leading the family in singing one of our old favorite songs.

I've thought about that moment a lot since then. There is real power in the music of our lives. I'm not sure I understand it, but there is something dramatic that happens when words and melodies mingle in our minds. It is burned into our consciousness. It becomes part of who we are and what we think—for good or ill—freezing moments in time.

Never to be forgotten.

JOSEPH WALKER

(Editor's note: This story appeared in The Ribbon *and in* Heartwarmers *in the summer of 2000.)*

The Victorian Tea Party

Today is my mother's eighty-sixth birthday, her first at the Michael G. Walsh Center; an Alzheimer's assisted living facility in Cleveland, Ohio. I have mixed emotions as I think of the Victorian tea party I've planned for this afternoon and how my mother will react.

The move had been traumatic. The "adjustment period" was well into its eighth month and our relationship was strained. The director of the Unit tried to reassure me that my mother was actively participating in group activities (meaning she is doing crafts, going out for lunch, etc.) and that she seemed happy. Since I was replenishing her petty cash fund, I believed this to be true; however, I didn't see it for myself.

My presence seemed to trigger a realization that her world had changed, that her daughter was visiting her in a place other than her own home, and that she missed something—what, she could not say. She often refused affection and instructed me: "Take me home where I belong." Visits usually ended with my husband, John, running interference or a staff member stepping in to distract mother while I walked away, choking back the tears.

1:15 p.m. John and I arrive at the Center. I'm carrying Mom's present—a sweater vest and matching slacks—which I hope will fit now that she's gained a bit of weight.

We take the elevator to the second floor. John enters the code that magically opens the double doors to the Unit. Resident suites line the brightly lit hallway. Everything is color coordinated and pleasing to the eye. The unit has a home-like feel: televisions blare, there's some activity in the kitchen, and the aroma of freshly brewed coffee permeates the air.

I'm greeted by one of the residents, a short, slender, gray-haired lady wearing a silk blouse, sweat pants, and bedroom slippers. "What's in the pretty box?"

"A birthday present for my mother, Ann Calabreeze."

"Is there going to be a party?" she asks, swaying back and forth in a child-like manner.

"Yes, and I hope you'll join us, Mrs. Crawford."

"Well, I haven't been invited!" (She pauses.) "Who is your mother?" She follows us down the hallway, stopping to talk with another resident. "Did you know there's a party?" Mr. Shoop dismisses her with a nod and walks back into his suite.

We head for the sunroom where Jodi, a staff member, is setting up for the party. She tells us Mom is resting in her room.

Lady Victoria, the woman I hired to present the program, is placing heirlooms: silks, laces, and delicate bouquets around the room. Two long tables border the windows, one for the sterling silver tea service, the other with ornate trays brimming with elegantly assorted finger sandwiches: chicken and almond, the Victorian cucumber sandwich, and fruited scones.

At the far end of the room, wearing a blue business suit and listening to the big band sound resounding from the tape recorder, is a new resident. The activity board propped near the fireplace reads:

Today is Monday, November 21, 1994
Clear, Sunny, 52 degrees
10 a.m.: Exercise
2 p.m.: Birthday Party

1:50 p.m. Residents are escorted to the sunroom. From a large box containing dozens of assorted hats, the women are invited to select a hat to wear to "tea." Crowned, these Queens for a Day proceed to their seats as the room takes on a sophisticated air of excitement.

"Is this only for ladies?" asks Mr. Cobb. He eyes the tray of finger sandwiches and smacks his lips. Jodi motions for him to have a seat by her, which he does, but not before grabbing a bowler hat and plopping it on his bald head. "How's that?" he chuckles. Some of the women laugh.

Lady Victoria, now wearing her fashionable raiment—a pink floor-length silk dress with bustle and a high collar, trimmed with black lace and topped with a matching regency hat—proceeds down the hallway to Mother's room. I follow. My mind reels back through past visits. *"Please, oh please, let today be different!"* I'm snapped back into the moment as Lady Victoria knocks, then opens Mom's door and calls, "Mrs. Calabreeze!"

"Yes?"

"Your daughter tells me it's your birthday today and *I am your present.*"

"Really?" Mom says in utter disbelief. She looks over at me, standing in the doorway, and smiles.

A sense of relief comes over me as I kiss her cheek. "I love you Mom. Happy Birthday!"

1-2-3-SURPRISE!

Mrs. Hoffichure, a robust lady in her early nineties, wearing a colorful housedress, hands Mom a flowered hat to wear; something like Jackie Kennedy would have worn (only without the flowers). The two of them join their friends seated at a nearby table and proceed to sample refreshments.

I sit behind them at a table with Mr. Shoop, who is quietly consuming one sandwich after another, and Mrs. Crawford, who can't decide if she should stay. "I didn't know there was a party today," she tells me. "I don't believe I was invited." I offer her a sandwich. "I don't want to impose," she says politely.

Out of nowhere, Mrs. Hoffichure points to my mother and bellows: "I love you in that hat, Jan!"

Mom giggles.

"I mean it! I *really* love you in that hat. Promise me you'll be buried in that hat, Jan!"

"Oh no!" Mother laughs out loud. Then turning to me, she whispers, "She thinks my name is Jan." We both smile.

Lady Victoria's program takes us back in time to an era of kings and queens. She talks about the language of the fans, calling card etiquette, and mourning traditions. As she speaks, I look around the room. Staff members are lovingly attending to residents. Mom and her friends seem to be into the program, frequently whispering "I had one of those" or "I remember that!" Some residents take mini-side trips into their own world, while others are busy tasting all the refreshments.

Marcia, Mother's afternoon caregiver, arrives as the program concludes. "Happy Birthday!" (She gives my mother a big hug and kiss.) "Did you have a good time?"

Mom gives her a warm smile, and with the innocence of a child replies, "Yes."

Taking that as our cue, John and I quietly leave.

It was a lovely party. Mom was happy, and in my heart I was happy, too, not only because everything went well, but also because my mother gave me a gift—the gift of understanding. Understanding that no matter how painful, we will get through this. An understanding that she has friends who care about her, that she lives in a place where she is treated with dignity, and where she is free to be herself. She has a life, and it is up to me to find my place.

LAVERN HALL

Generation to Generation

As the old woman reclines in her wheelchair, staring vacantly into space, no longer speaking or feeding herself, you wonder why God allows her to live.

"What is her life worth?" people ask me about my mother.

Then I watch as the two-year-old runs across the room and touches her hand. His six-year-old sister holds up a picture she's drawn and says, "See what I made for you, Grandma DeeDee."

With effort the old lady focuses on them and smiles. When the little boy sits in the chair beside her, she rubs his soft hair. The little girl gives her a hug. She can't use words to communicate with the children but the sense of love surrounds them.

Tears come to my eyes as I watch the generations respond to one another, in a world where age and recognition don't matter. My grandchildren and my mother share through their smiles and through touch.

❦   ❦   ❦

Mother Has a Purpose
"She has a purpose," I say to myself. "She is touching the lives of her great-grandchildren and teaching them about family relationships and caring, even though she doesn't realize it. God has a purpose for her life and a reason, it seems, for her to

continue living, even though it's not the type of life we would desire if conditions were ideal."

❧   ❧   ❧

Ravages of Alzheimer's
My mother has Alzheimer's disease and has been in a nursing home for more than six years. She no longer knows who I am, or if she does, it's in fleeting glimpses. She can't feed herself nor care for herself.

But she does respond to touch and kind words with her lovely smile.

My grandchildren, two-year-old Alex and six-year-old Kara, accompany me on weekly visits. They seem to enjoy these trips to the nursing home and seeing Great Grandma DeeDee and the other residents. Alex doesn't understand who she is; but apparently she's become a familiar face to him because he'll pick her out in a room of residents and run to her wheelchair. Kara knows that Great Grandma no longer can care for herself and requires more attention than we can give at home.

❧   ❧   ❧

Children Enjoy the Nursing Home
Both children also enjoy participating in special events at the nursing home—Christmas and New Year's parties, an Easter egg hunt, and sharing these occasions with family members. They also like to be involved in activities, such as bingo, exercise class, and crafts.

❧   ❧   ❧

Families Can Participate

Placing a relative in a nursing home may not be the way we would wish to handle the situation if conditions were ideal. But life usually doesn't hand us perfect situations. We must consider the realities and act accordingly.

However, we can still experience interaction as a family unit. We can teach our children and grandchildren that the elderly are important and need our attention. The children also learn that family members have varying degrees of capability and require different kinds of care and love.

❧   ❧   ❧

Not Depressing for Children

"I think it's so depressing for children to see old people like that," I've been told.

However, my grandchildren don't feel that way. To them it's fun to visit the nursing home. They can make Great Grandma DeeDee smile, receive attention from the other residents and staff, draw pictures for Great Grandma and other residents, and have a tea party with Great Grandma. To them, being old is a natural part of life and going to visit Great Grandma at the nursing home will be remembered with pleasure and fondness.

"And we make Grandma DeeDee happy," concludes Kara, when asked why she visits a woman who doesn't know her.

"Grandma smiles," comments Alex, and his face breaks into a wide grin.

"Grandma happy."

They reveal that enjoyment is a two-way relationship as they interact with their great-grandmother and form a bond of love between the generations.

※ ※ ※

I wrote this two years ago. My mother is still alive and even less capable. However, visiting her at the nursing home still delights Kara and Alex. They hope I'll time my visits for the hours they're out of school so they can accompany me.

MARY EMMA ALLEN
Author and Speaker

(Editor's note: This story appeared in Straight from the Heart *and* The Ribbon *in the winter of 2000.)*

A Golden Retriever Makes a Difference

During a visit to a county facility, we were told of a woman by the name of Katie. She suffered from dementia and had not spoken a word in seven years.

The recreational therapist thought that perhaps a visit from Katie, a golden retriever, would be helpful.

Upon entering her room the therapist said to Katie, "This is Katie."

The woman took that golden head into her hands, looked deep into those beautiful, liquid-brown eyes, and stated clearly and without hesitation, "Katie, you are a golden retriever."

You can well imagine the shock from the facility's staff.

A therapy dog had reached into that quiet, lonely place, and for a moment, Katie had Katie.

KATHY TERRY
Tester/Observer, Therapy Dogs, Inc.

A Hug, A Tender Touch

They only need a moment,
That's not asking very much.
Just give them each a greeting,
A hug, a tender touch.

Stroke the greying lock of hair.
Or kiss the weathered cheek,
And go about your business,
Your full and busy week.

It won't take long to visit.
They have nothing
    much to say.
Their days are pretty
    much the same
But pause along the way,

And join them in their world,
For just a little while.
Long enough to greet them,
Long enough to make them
    smile.

There's no longer very many
Who take time out of their
    day

To concern themselves about
    them.
It's too depressing, so they say.

They are diapered, and they
    slobber,
And they dribble at their food
They may not talk
    intelligently
Or be in a happy mood,

But spare a smile, a tender
    touch,
Knowledge that they exist,
For there may be a point
    in time
When you end up like this.

When your loved ones will
    forsake you
Cause you won't know
    they are there,
But you need a hug from
    someone,
You need someone there to
    care.

MARIAN SUMMERS

Contributors' Biographies

Mary Emma ALLEN is the author of *When We Become the Parent to Our Parents,* her mother's journey through Alzheimer's. She is a columnist, children's storywriter, and book author. Mary Emma gives talks to nursing homes and to groups about coping with this disease. Visit her website at: http://alzheimersnotes. blogspot.com. Send Mary Emma an e-mail at: me.allen@juno.com

Mary S. BARRASS has a BS in Computer Information Systems and is working on her Master's Degree. She is a Corporate Lead Auditor at a major medical device facility in Northridge, California. She lives in Lancaster, California with her good friend and adopted mother, Evelyn Daniel. Mary is a widow and lost her twenty-two-year-old son, Mark, as well as her father, mother, sister, and brother.

Diane BLAKE writes, "In late 1999, I moved my eighty-eight-year-old mother from her home in Chicago to our home in California. Since then, I have discovered a previously untapped well of patience within myself! Caring for my mother has reinforced the adage: *Once an adult; twice a child.*"

Rosa Lee BOSLAR worked for thirty years and raised four children. She now enjoys retirement and spoiling her grandchildren.

Dr. Marlene CAROSELLI has authored fifty-five books (see Amazon.com). She also keynotes and conducts corporate training. She can be reached via e-mail at mccpd@frontiernet.net, by phone at 1-585-249-0084, or through her website www.caroselli.biz.

Debbie CENTER has lived in Littleton, Colorado, for thirty-one years. She stays at home with her two children and teaches piano in her home. She also plays professionally. Ms. Center writes, "I would love to hear from other people dealing with dementia in their parents, especially if anyone has experienced the visual agnosia that Mom has. My e-mail address is pianomam@aol.com."

Evelyn DANIEL, widow of Donald Daniel, who succumbed to Alzheimer's disease, attended Central State College (Edmond, Oklahoma) and the University of Oklahoma–Norman. Published: *Essays to Myself, Keep Doing it Until You Get it Right,* and *Dialogues with Donald.*

Sharon DeMOE writes, "My husband and I live in Oklahoma. We have a wonderful, supportive, and loving family, which includes our two daughters, two sons-in-law and four terrific granddaughters. Thank you all—family and friends near and far, for the love you have shown to Jerry and me. And thank you Brenda, for giving me this opportunity to share my story."

Laurie FRASIER is her son's mom, her four stepchildren's mom, her mom's mom, and a wife. She works in a Child Advocacy Center when she is not with her family. She lives in Grand Junction, Colorado where she devotes her life to family, fun, and adventure.

Joan FRY's short stories, celebrity interviews, and human-interest articles have appeared in *Reader's Digest, Los Angeles Times, Other Voices, Black Warrior Review, Westways, Practical Horseman,* and countless other national publications. A horse lover, she co-authored *The Beginning Dressage Book* and lives with her husband, her mother-in-law, and her horse in Acton, California.

Lavern HALL, RN, MA, has cared for three family members during the past twelve years. She is the editor/publisher of *A Glass Full of Tears: Dementia Day-by-Day,* a book helpful to caregivers and healthcare professionals. Excerpts have been published in two Houghton-Mifflin textbooks. Contact her at Writer's World Press, 35 N. Chillicothe Road, Aurora, Ohio 44202 or WritersWorld@juno. com.

Caleb Stephen JORDAN writes, "I am ten years old—will be eleven on April 20, 2001, and I am in 5th grade at Lincoln Orchard Mesa Elementary School. I reside in Grand Junction, Colorado. It has been a pleasure writing for this book and I really hope that you enjoy it."

Micah J. LESLIE, an attorney and corporate executive, emphatically states his proudest achievements come from his role as caregiver for his dementia-stricken mother. As a tribute to his mother, Micah has produced an Alzheimer's CD titled *We Can Make A Difference,* a compilation of eleven original songs to touch the hearts of those on this journey of continuing good-byes.

Cindy LESTER is the Adult Respite Coordinator of the Daybreak program—a cooperative effort between the Kenosha Area Family & Aging Services, Inc. and the Kenosha County Division of Aging Services. Cindy resides in Salem, Wisconsin with her husband and two children. Her background is in Oncology Rehabilitative Services, Assistant Nursing, and Alzheimer's/Dementia Care. She feels blessed to work with the participants that bring her "JOY" every day!

Linda (L2Photoljt@aol.com) is from the Midwest and now lives in California. Her father was diagnosed in February 1997. Linda says, "*The Gathering Place-Online Alzheimer's Caregiver Support* evolved since I cannot help my family directly. I may never meet those who are helped, but as they 'gather' information, they will be able to continue to 'pay it forward' to someone else in search of help."

Gil LOZANO was born and raised in Los Angeles and educated in Southern California. After thirty-five years with Rockwell International he retired in 1995. Caring for his late mother, after his father passed away in 1987, Gil continued to play an active role in her care after she was admitted into an Alzheimer's facility.

A. Nony MOUS prefers to go by his middle name.

Jeanne PARSONS retired after working as a psychiatric technician and as an emergency room surgical assistant. She says she could not have cared for her mother for seven years without the help of her daughter, Julie Sullivan and part-time caregiver, Sarphine Phillips. Jeanne wrote these stories with the help of her wonderful friend Viola B. Good.

Marion RILEY writes, "Don and I were married on May 19, 1946 in Troy, New York. We have five children. In 1954 we moved to California, where we enjoyed many happy years and saw our family grow and give us fourteen grandchildren and eight great-grandchildren."

Kay RUNNER, a resident of Lancaster, California since 1955, raised four children and now enjoys spending time with her nine grandchildren. Kay is active with the Visiting Nurse Adult Day Care Program Advisory Council, Lancaster First Baptist Church, and the Antelope Valley Republican Assembly. Since the death of her mother

(March 1999) and her husband (June 1999), she devotes her time to these activities as they bring her much joy.

Jonathan SCHULKIN In September 1996, when Elizabeth's condition deteriorated, the Schulkins moved from Florida to Lancaster, California to be closer to their daughter, a resident of Ventura, California. Now retired from real estate development and sales, Mr. Schulkin keeps active with visiting his wife, volunteer work, and church activities.

Marian SUMMERS is the proud mother of three children: two daughters living in Arizona, and a son in Kansas. She is at home in Lincoln, Nebraska where for the last year her husband, Ronald, has been a patient at the Tabitha Health Care Center in the final stages of Alzheimer's.

Kathy TERRY has been volunteering with Therapy Dogs, Inc. since 1992. Kathy has been a Tester/Observer with TD, Inc. since 1994, introducing many people to the concept of animal-assisted therapy—with its tears and abundant joys. May those who read these stories be moved to join forces with animal-assisted therapy.

Joseph WALKER, a freelance writer and editor, writes a nationally syndicated newspaper column called "ValueSpeak" and edits *Pioneer* magazine for the Sons of Utah Pioneers. His published books include, *How Can You Mend A Broken Spleen?* and *The Mission: Inside The Church of Jesus Christ of Latter-day Saints.* Joseph and his wife, Anita, are parents of five children. They reside in American Fork, Utah.

Loraine YATES asks simply to be known as "Caregiver for My Little Mama." It is her heartfelt wish to help others through her writing.

Eula YOUNGBLOOD is a Licensed Vocational Nurse with a BA in Business and a BS in Mechanical Engineering. She studied teleplay writing for seven years in the Los Angeles Open Door Program (auspices of Writer's Guild of America West) and received an Honorable Mention in their Annual Writers' Competition in 1975. While employed in Quality Management for twenty-five years, Eula wrote a number of accepted teleplays and stage plays.

Updated contributors' biographies (2006)

Resources and Programs

Alzheimer's Association

225 North Michigan Avenue, 17th Floor Chicago, IL 60611
Tel: 1-800-272-3900 Website: www.alz.org

A network of state and local chapters, this is the largest national voluntary health organization committed to finding a cure for Alzheimer's and helping those affected by the disease. Call for support group information and to find the chapter nearest you. See below for information on Memories in the Making™ and the Safe Return Program.

Alzheimer's Disease Education and Referral (ADEAR)

P.O. Box 8250, Silver Spring, MD 20907-8250
Tel: 1-800-438-4380 Website: www.alzheimers.org/org

Information about Alzheimer's disease and related disorders. The ADEAR Center is a service of the National Institute on Aging (NIA). NIA News: Research on Alzheimer's Disease Website: http://www.alzheimers.org/nianews/nianews.html

Alzheimer's Foundation of America (AFA)

322 8th Ave., 6th Fl., New York, NY 10001
Tel: 1-866-232-8484 Website: www.alzfdn.org/

Provide optimal care and services to individuals confronting dementia, and to their caregivers and families—through member organizations dedicated to improving quality of life.

American Health Assistance Foundation (AHAF)

22512 Gateway Center Drive, Clarksburg, Maryland 20871
Tel: 1-800-437-2423 Website: www.ahaf.org

A nonprofit charitable organization with over thirty years dedicated to funding research on Alzheimer's disease, glaucoma, macular degeneration, heart disease, and stroke; educating the public about these diseases; and providing financial assistance to Alzheimer's disease patients and their caregivers.

Eldercare Locator
Tel: 1-800-677-1116   1-202-872-0888
Website: www.n4a.org
A free nationwide directory assistance service to help older persons and caregivers locate local support resources. Administered through the National Association of Area Agencies on Aging in Washington, D.C.

ElderCare Online—Internet Community of Elder Caregivers
Website: www.ec-online.net/Community/Neighborhood/neighbor-hood.html
ElderCare Online's Neighborhood Network contains links to state, county, and local resources, including Alzheimer's disease support groups and Area Agencies on Aging.

Memories in the Making™
Tel: 1-949-955-9000
This signature art program of the Alzheimer's Association of Orange County, helps improve the quality of life for people suffering from Alzheimer's disease. When words fail, art allows the individual with Alzheimer's another way to communicate feelings.

National Family Caregivers Association (NFCA)
10400 Connecticut Ave., Ste. 500, Kensington, MD 20895-3944
Tel: 1-301-942-6430 1-800-896-3650
E-mail: info@nfcacares.org Website: www.nfcacares.org
The NFCA is a grassroots organization created to educate, support, empower, and speak up for the millions of Americans who care for chronically ill, aged, or disabled loved ones. Inquire about free membership for family caregivers.

Safe Return Program
The Alzheimer's Association's nationwide program that assists in the identification and safe and timely return of people with Alzheimer's disease and related disorders who wander. See "Alzheimer's Association" for contact information.

Updated resources and programs (2006)

Suggested Reading/Listening

Avadian, Brenda, MA, ed. *Finding the JOY in Alzheimer's-Vol. 2: When Tears are Dried with Laughter.* Lancaster, CA: North Star Books, 2003.

Avadian, Brenda, MA *"Where's my shoes?" My Father's Walk Through Alzheimer's (2nd ed.).* Pearblossom, CA: North Star Books, 2005.

Avadian, Brenda, MA (author) and Barbara Caruso (narrator). *"Where's my shoes?" My Father's Walk Through Alzheimer's (1st ed).* Unabridged audio book. Prince Frederick: Recorded Books, LLC, 2000.

Bell, Virginia and David Troxel, MPHS. *The Best Friends Approach to Alzheimer's Care.* Baltimore: Health Professions Press, 2003.

Brackey, Jolene. *Creating Moments of Joy for the Person with Alzheimer's or Dementia: A Journal for Caregivers.* West Lafayette: Purdue University Press, 2000.

Feil, Naomi. *The Validation Breakthrough: Simple Techniques for Communicating with People with "Alzheimer's-Type Dementia" (2nd ed.).* Baltimore: Health Professions Press, 2002.

FitzRay, B.J. *Alzheimer's Activities: Hundreds of Activities for Men and Women with Alzheimer's Disease and Related Disorders.* Windsor: Rayve Productions, 2001.

Hardship into Hope: The Rewards of Caregiving. (Audiocassette). Connie Goldman Productions, 1999. 926 Second Street, Suite 201, Santa Monica, CA 90403. Tel: 310-393-6801 E-mail: congoldman@aol.com

Mace, Nancy L., MA and Peter V. Rabins, MD, MPH. *The 36-Hour Day: A Family Guide to Caring for Persons with Alzheimer's Disease, Related Dementing Illnesses, and Memory Loss in Later Life.* (Revised Edition). New York: Warner Books, 2001.

Peterson, Betsy. *Voices of Alzheimer's: Courage, Humor, Hope, and Love in the Face of Dementia.* Cambridge: DeCapo Press, 2004.

TheCaregiversVoice.com—Gives a voice to the millions of caregivers who care for their loved ones. Access this site for news updates, links to other informative sites, and to submit your stories for the *Finding the JOY* series of books., P.O. Box 589, Pearblossom, CA 93553-0589 Tel: 661-944-1130 Website: www.TheCaregivers-Voice.com

The Ribbon—free online newsletter for families and caregivers dealing with Alzheimer's disease and other dementias. Subscribe online at Website: www.TheRibbon.com, or by mail at *The Ribbon,* 1325 Venus Drive, Nashville, TN 37217-1918.

Today's Caregiver—the first national magazine dedicated to caregivers. Caregiver Media Group, 6365 Taft Street, Suite 3006, Hollywood, FL 33024. Tel: 800-829-2734 Website: www.Caregiver.com

Updated suggested reading/listening list (2006)

154 ❦

Permissions continued from page 4

CareGiver. Printed with permission from Loraine Yates. ©1999 Loraine Yates

A Child Shows the Way. Reprinted with permission from Mary Emma Allen. ©2000 Mary Emma Allen

Dave Ferguson. Photo courtesy of Lockheed Martin. ©1990

"Damn, you're handsome!" Printed with permission from Micah Leslie. ©1999 Micah Leslie

"Do I have Erectile Dysfunction?" Based on a story by Gil Lozano. ©1999 Gil Lozano

Don't Eat the Yellow and Green Ones. Printed with permission from Loraine Yates. ©2000 Loraine Yates

"Do you take...in sickness and in health?" "I do." Printed with permission from Sharon DeMoe. ©2001 Sharon DeMoe

Dreams Swept In. Printed with permission from Evelyn Daniel. ©1999 Evelyn Daniel

Family of Friends. Signed permission form on file.

Four Generations of the Lozano Family. Photo courtesy of Gil Lozano. ©2000

Four Special Days. Printed with permission from Laurie Frasier. ©2000 Laurie Frasier

Generation to Generation. Reprinted with permission from Mary Emma Allen. ©2000 Mary Emma Allen

A Golden Retriever Makes a Difference. Printed with permission from Kathy Terry. ©1999 Kathy Terry

Good Things Out of Bad. Printed with permission from Caleb Stephen Jordan. ©2000 Caleb Stephen Jordan

A Hug, A Tender Touch. Printed with permission from Marian Summers. ©2000 Marian Summers

Ice Cream Never Tasted So Good. Printed with permission from Debbie Center. ©2001 Debbie Center

"I forget dear, what's an orgasm?" Printed with permission from Jeanne Parsons. ©2001 Jeanne Parsons

Is it C.R.S. or Alzheimer's? Printed with permission from Eula Youngblood. ©2001 Eula Youngblood

"I've got rocks in my head!" Printed with permission from Loraine Yates. ©1999 Loraine Yates

Lovers for Fifty-Six Years. Printed with permission from Evelyn Daniel. ©1999 Evelyn Daniel

Martin Avadian hamming it up for the camera. Photos courtesy of David Borden. ©1999

"May I help you?" Signed permission form on file.

The Naked Bride. Printed with permission from Marlene Caroselli. ©1999 Marlene Caroselli

Never to be Forgotten. Reprinted with permission from Joseph Walker. ©2000 Joseph Walker

A Prayer Answered. Excerpt from *Dialogues with Donald.* Reprinted with permission from Mary Barrass. ©2000 Mary Barrass

Slept Right Through Thanksgiving. Printed with permission from Kay Runner. ©2001 Kay Runner

Sonny Sagas. Printed with permission from Rosa Lee Boslar. ©2001 Rosa Lee Boslar

Those Three Words. Printed with permission from Jonathan Schulkin. ©2001 Jonathan Schulkin

The Victorian Tea Party. Printed with permission from Lavern Hall. ©2000 Lavern Hall

The Wedding. Printed with permission from Cindy Lester. ©2001 Cindy Lester

"What's the name of that disease where you forget...?" Printed with permission from Diane Blake. ©1999 Diane Blake

Whose Prosthesis is This Anyway? Printed with permission from Gil Lozano. ©1998 Gil Lozano

About the Author

Brenda Avadian, MA, cared for her father until he passed away from Alzheimer's at age ninety. While others worry and express hopelessness, Brenda tries to find the humor in life's challenges and helps fellow caregivers do the same.

Brenda is the author of eight books, including the *Finding the JOY* series designed to uplift and raise awareness. When only a handful of family caregivers were talking about their experiences, Brenda authored the pioneering caregiver's memoir, *"Where's my shoes?" My Father's Walk Through Alzheimer's*—now available in a fully revised and expanded second edition.

Brenda's passion, enthusiasm, and tireless efforts to help caregivers are why many organizations invite her to speak about caring for people with Alzheimer's.

Prior to becoming a caregiver, Brenda coached members of the corporate world toward becoming better leaders and communicators. She also taught at the University of Wisconsin-Milwaukee, Marquette University, Alverno College, and co-designed and facilitated Lockheed's executive development program at the University of Southern California. In 1989, she was commissioned a Kentucky Colonel for her contributions to public service. Since 1998, she has served as an award-winning member of Toastmasters International.

Born in Milwaukee, Wisconsin, Brenda earned her bachelor's and master's degrees from the University of Wisconsin-Milwaukee. She met her husband, David Borden, in Milwaukee. They live with their orange tabby cat on five acres near the Angeles National Forest in Los Angeles.

Sales proceeds of Brenda's books are donated worldwide.

Updated author biography (2006)

Submit Your JOYFUL Caregiving Story

Do you have a JOYFUL story about caring for a loved one with brain impairment or dementia caused by Alzheimer's, stroke, related illness, or trauma?

Do you have a photo or artwork of a JOYFUL time with a loved one with a brain-impairing illness or disease?

Dear Caregiver:

I invite you to submit your work for consideration in **Finding the JOY in Caregiving**—the third volume of our **Finding the JOY** series.

Submission Guidelines are online at www.TheCaregiversVoice.com (click on the **Community** tab)

Together we will bring hope and JOY to caregivers!

Genuinely Yours,

Brenda Avadian, MA

Order Information

Please ask for our titles at your neighborhood bookstore, library, or buy them at an online retailer.

You may also support The Caregiver's Voice by purchasing books at www.TheCaregiversVoice.com (click on the **Products & Services** tab).

Finding the JOY
in Alzheimer's:
Caregivers Share
the JOYFUL Times

Finding the JOY
in Alzheimer's:
When Tears are
Dried with Laughter

"Where's my shoes?"
My Father's Walk through Alzheimer's

To order VOLUME copies contact:

NORTH STAR BOOKS
P.O. Box 589 • Pearblossom, CA 93553
Telephone: 661.944.1130
E-mail: NSB@NorthStarBooks.com

CPSIA information can be obtained
at www.ICGtesting.com
Printed in the USA
FFOW03n1145020118
44291567-43867FF